What Doctors Didn't Tell Us

About Double Breasted Suits and Single Breasted Women

By

Martha Falterman & Neppie Trahan & Loretta Schultz

ISBN: 0-7596-7066-8

This book is printed on acid free paper.

1stBooks – rev. 02/27/02

Table of Contents

iii

Martha's Story

Since my initial diagnosis in April 1993, I have had five biopsies (three breast and two endometrium biopsies) and have had two skin cancers removed from my back (too much sun as a child). I heard somewhere "only 15% of the time it is malignant and the other 85% of the time it is benign." In my case, this is definitely true. Only the first internal biopsy was malignant.

Someone once said that I should write about my bout with cancer. At first I wondered why - doesn't everyone go through the same thing? Have I really been dealt a bad hand? You be the judge, my story begins here.

While taking a shower one night, getting ready to go to a singles party, I decided to do a self-breast exam. I had wet hands and my breasts were wet. I examined the left breast - fine. Then the right breast - Oh, no! It can't be! Oh S——-! There was a lump that I could put between my fingers. It was so large it felt like a marble. Think positive - shower, dry, and reexamine. Upon reexamination it felt even larger. What do I do? It's Saturday afternoon - whom do I call? Play like it's not there and don't worry until Monday. After all, it could go away.

God can't try me like this! Three weeks prior to being diagnosed with cancer, I had quit smoking. After all I had quit smoking several times before this and had always returned to it because of the weight I would gain. How could I go through this and not smoke. Weight was only a minor problem. This was my life.

I went to the party that night and a few friends commented that I was unusually quiet. I said it was the stress of no nicotine, so the natural thing to do was smoke. I bummed one and it tasted horrible but I didn't put it out. Then I felt guilty. No, I'm not going to smoke. Put it out - the end.

The next week I called and the first obstacle was to get an appointment with my gynecologist. After I explain the circumstances I am given an appointment for Thursday afternoon. How can I go that long without a cigarette? Keep busy. I go to work (teaching math at a middle school), exercise for 2 ½ hours instead of just 1½ hours, and take an Excedrin PM nightly.

Thursday arrives and D-Day is here. The technician tries not to alarm me, but goes to get the radiologist. He examines me, and then asks me to dress and follow him. We go to the room where x-rays are viewed and there it is. It looks like a ball with antenna and feelers growing from it. It looks like something from outer space. I can remember saying, "I'm not a doctor, but this doesn't look good!" He responds, "No, it doesn't!"

How could this be happening? I had a mammogram each year for eleven years. Nothing. I had a mammogram eight months before. Nothing. I go to church regularly. I know people who don't. I know people who steal and others who cheat on their spouses. They don't develop cancer - Why Me? It's just not fair! I'm single and teach school for a living - I can't afford to be sick! My only child, a daughter, is sixteen years old and living with her Dad in another part of the state, we have to develop a better relationship. This is not fair - it's just NOT FAIR!!!!

The next step is the surgeon. I had been told that if you look carefully into Dr. Breaux's eyes while he is examining you, his expression changes if he feels it is something to be concerned about. I watched his face carefully and did notice that dreaded change. Another hope washed away. Things are not going my way. He agrees to do the biopsy the next day.

Now, I must tell my parents. They are both in their late 70's. How do I do this? I must be strong! They have taught me this - keep face. I call and my Mom starts chit chatting, I let her talk, and then ask for Daddy to get on the other phone. I said, "I have something to tell you, and I only want to say it one time."

She pauses, and summons Dad to get on the other phone. She had no clue what to expect. Last time I spoke like that I told them I was walking out of my marriage with a 7-year-old child. What could Martha be up to now?

After relaying the events of the previous two weeks I explained that I was going the next day for a biopsy only. I had already made plans for my younger sister, Robin, to drive me to the hospital at 5:30 A. M. I tell them not to worry; I'll call when it's all over. Pause. Silence. My Dad says OK and Mom is speechless. I chit chat and hang up. Oh Lord, Lelia (Mom) is going for a Valium and Jules (Dad) for a scotch! (The day after I wrote this part I was talking to my Mom, she looked at me and said, "It was a Butosol, not a Valium.")

Prior to calling my parents I had called my brother, J.E., and told him I was going to break the news to them. J.E. had been consoling me for two weeks and I knew he would do the same for my parents. He just kept saying, "Martha, Daddy has those lymphoma's all over his body. I bet it's no more than that!" Somehow, those words had kept me from losing my mind for the past two weeks.

5:00 A.M. - can't drink coffee, can't drink water - I'm a nervous wreck!!! Call Ask-A-Nurse - Yes, I can chew gum. Arrive at Our Lady of Lourdes Medical Center, dress in hospital attire, start the IV, watch TV - what else?

Around 8:30 A.M. my parents arrive. Somehow I knew they would come and yet I wanted to spare the pain that this would cause. They don't need this stress at this stage of life. The nurses, anesthesiologists, etc. come to the room periodically and say it will be a while longer, yet no one will give me an idea of when.

At 2:30 P.M. they finally come to get me. Smiles are exchanged and I begin to cry. I'm so scared. My family is there, yet I feel so alone. One more look at them. They, too, have tears in their eyes.

Biopsy performed. When I come to in recovery I ask the nurses for the results. Each gives the same response, "I don't know - I'm just a recovery nurse." Shortly afterwards they roll me back to my room.

My Mom, my Dad, and Robin are just looking at me - each with a long, fearful face. "Do I have Cancer?" I asked. "Oh, don't worry, you're young, you can do It." were the first words out of my Dad's mouth. I look at my Mom, "Do I have Cancer?"

"We're here for you, don't worry about a thing! You're a young, healthy woman!" she says.

I look at Robin, "Please tell me. Do I have Cancer?"

"Yes, Martha, you do!"

My God, I'll never forget those words. I begin to cry.

My Dad looked at me and I could see he wanted to comfort me, yet didn't know how. He said, "Don't cry. It's going to be

OK." "Let me cry! Let me get it out! Then I'm going to figure out how to fight this!"

A little while later Dr. Breaux came to the room, and again said those dreaded words, "I'm sorry to tell you this, but you have breast cancer. You and I talked lumpectomy yesterday, but that will be impossible. I **saw** too much cancer. It will be necessary for me to perform a mastectomy."

I looked at him and the first words out of my mouth, "I have a 16- year-old daughter I need to see grow up. I can do that without a right breast." All of a sudden my life's priorities changed and I really understood that old saying, *"When you have your health, you have everything."* Easter Week is here (I have to wait another week for the surgery) and I am really stressing. My daughter, Toni, comes to Lafayette and we have a wonderful time. I talk openly and honestly about cancer and tell her I am not giving up hope. I will fight this with the last breath in my body.

Sunday afternoon I send her back to her Dad's and assure her that I will have someone call when I am out of surgery, Tuesday. As she is driving away tears are flowing down my face, cheeks, neck - I hate all of this uncertainty. Who is going to help me? I'm alone. What's going to happen to me?

The next day I go on extended sick leave, the last six weeks of school, turn in my keys and grade book, and walk away from

Judice Middle School with tears in my eyes. These kids have been looking at me and they don't know what to say. So are the teachers and other staff members. I smiled and assured them that I would make it. Then I turn away and cry. Can I continue to pretend to be so strong?

Several years prior to being diagnosed with cancer I had experienced one of those "joys of life" HA! - A divorce. A priest used to say, "Crying purges the soul. It looks like Martha has been purged again." I need to call him and let him know the purging process is working overtime.

Tuesday is here. I'm packed for the hospital. Do I have everything? The standard supplies are there (toothbrush, toothpaste, face wash, etc.) No, I won't need make up. Yes, button down the front pajamas and robe. (I've been told I won't be able to raise my arm for a while). OK. D-Day is here.

I arrive at Our Lady of Lourdes Medical Center around 5:30 A.M., dressed in one of those designer hospital gowns, and begin the process of being rolled from room to room. My sister, Robin, has been so kind, again, to get up early and help me. She is truly a jewel!

Surgery goes well and I wake up in recovery. Shortly afterward I arrive in my room. Upon opening my eyes the first thing I see is a lovely potted plant my Dad had brought. He knows I love flowers and he wanted to make sure that I had

7

these. My Mom, Dad, and Robin are in the room. They look worried, but relieved this first step is over.

Family, friends, co-workers, other breast cancer survivors all come by to let me know they are thinking about me and praying that the outcome will be good. This is reassuring. All these flowers are nice, but prayers will help the most.

The second day at home I decided it was time for me to face reality. I needed to see for myself that my breast was gone and what I looked like. I stand in front of a mirror and unbutton my shirt; the first things I see are two drainage bags filling with blood. Then I lift the gauze placed over the incision. Staples are perfectly placed from my breastbone to under my arm. Oh God! This is so ugly. My left breast looks smaller than ever and nothing on the right side. Oh God - is this what I'm going to look like? I don't know if I can handle this! While in front of that mirror, the phone rings. It was Dr. Breaux's nurse. She was inquiring as to how I am doing. She can sense that I have been crying and she asks more questions. It was then that I told her of what I had done.

"It's a little soon for you to be looking. Why did you do it now?" she asks.

"It's not going to go away. I needed to look."

I have always felt that I was the type of person who could fight anything, as long as I knew what I was fighting. This action affirmed this. From here on I will fight CANCER even more. It may get me "down", but it will not be my doom. One slogan that I have lived by is *"The greatest thing in this world is not where we are, but in what direction we are moving"*. I decided that day at age 45, I was to move ahead full force and make the best of this "nasty C" that is in my body. Fight! Fight! Fight!

A few days later Dr. Breaux calls; he had received the pathology report. He informs me that thirty-six lymph nodes were removed and **thirteen** were **positive**. At that point these are just numbers. I assume everyone has them. It wasn't for several months, after researching and talking to other survivors, that I realized that my case was very serious.

The oncologist I chose to see is Dr. Paulette Blanchet. God steered me in the right direction. She has truly been wonderful. It was decided that I would have eight chemo treatments, each three weeks apart. (Damn, I had planned to finish before school started in the fall. I guess God had planned differently). This means six months of chemo and six weeks of radiation. I'll finish all this mess at the end of the year. God, forgive me, but I'm going to really plan a New Year's celebration this year.

After talking to Dr. Blanchet I am made aware that my hair will fall out after my first treatment, but she assures me that it will grow back. OK. The first thing I do is cut my shoulder length hair short because it's less traumatic for short hair to fall out, get a wig, and then get a mediport (another one-day surgery). The mediport is what will be used to administer the chemotherapy treatments. A cranial prosthesis is the medical name for a wig. The insurance company will not pay for a "wig." They consider it an unnecessary medical expense.

Ready, set, go! Start that chemo! When the first treatment was begun, tears were involuntarily streaming down. I didn't want to go through this. I didn't want to start it. I didn't want to lose my hair. I don't want to get fat. About thirty minutes into the first treatment the tears subside. I remember those words Fight! Fight! Fight! And that's what I'm going to do.

I had heard many horror stories of chemo and I was so afraid. Believe me. It's not that bad. I was never nauseated, never had diarrhea. My biggest problem was I could not keep my head up - I slept all day and night for the first forty-eight hours. Then when I woke up, I couldn't sleep. If that's the worse that I get - I can live with this.

First treatment completed and I'm waiting for my hair to fall, and it doesn't. Second treatment down and a few days later I'm invited to an end of the year school party. I'm feeling good so I go to be with my fiends. I place my fingers in the back of my head, and when I remove them, hair is in my hand. I make an excuse and leave the party quickly. While driving home I put a crack in my window, remove hair from head, and let it blow in the wind. That night while taking a shower, I washed my hair (my scalp was itching) and it fell out in handfuls, yet there was still hair on my head. The water wouldn't drain from the tub because the drain was clogged with my hair. It was really depressing to have to remove my own hair from the tub. When I woke up the next morning hair was all over my pillow and sheets, yet there was still some on my head. At that point I called my beautician and asked for a Sinead O'Connor (she had just torn up a picture of the Pope on Saturday Night Live and everyone in this Catholic community knew about her!) Now when I washed my scalp and my hair fell, the hair could go down the drain. Instead of the hair controlling my feelings, I took the lead and controlled it. Now it could fall, but was so ugly it didn't matter. For the next ten months a cranial prosthesis and scarves would be my best friends. I only wore scarves around my house. The wig would give me a feeling of being almost normal when I went out in public. (If you are a cancer patient reading this, I suggest you get a wig while you still have hair on your head. You can match the color much better.)

Chemo treatments continue May, June, July and no major problems. After having an extended summer I am really looking forward to going back to work. I go to school early and begin getting my room together slowly. (My energy level is not what it had been prior to April.) School starts and all is well. The second week of school I come home, put on my workout clothes and am planning to go to Red's Health Club to walk the air-conditioned indoor track. When I raise my left leg to tie my tennis shoe, I feel something strange in my left breast. Immediately I begin to do a self-breast exam and my worse nightmare is revealed. I feel a lump that I can place between my two fingers. It moves. Remove the bra - check again - this can't be real. Yes! It is! Stay calm or at least pretend. How can this be happening to me? I haven't got a strand of hair on my head, I'm on chemo, and I'm finding a lump in the other breast. This isn't fair - it isn't fair.

I can't tell my parents yet. I decide I will wait and maybe they won't need to know about this scare I'm having. I make an appointment to see Dr. Breaux, my surgeon.

While he is examining my breast I look carefully for that change in his facial expression. Maybe I won't see it this time. No such luck. It's there again! He questions me about my chemo and I tell him I'm taking Adriamycin, Cytoxan, and 5-FU. He again has a puzzled look. Then he says, "I'm going to have to do a biopsy and I'll need for you to sign giving permission for me to do a mastectomy if it is malignant. I'll try not to have to remove your mediport."

Now the tears are streaming down my face and I can't stop. All I could say was, "This isn't fair! It's just not fair! I don't have a lick of hair on my head and now you're telling me my cancer could be spreading. I'm not trained in medicine, but I know this is not good. Oh S——! I don't know how much of this I can take." At that point the nurse excused herself, she was crying. I was talking and crying. Dr. Breaux just stayed with me trying to calm me down. He stayed with me for what seemed like a long time; then, I dressed and was walking out of the office. I stopped to pay for my visit and even the receptionist was straining to keep from crying. I'm numb - What next?

Again I have to tell my parents that I will undergo another biopsy. I wait until the last minute to call and just state it as a matter of fact that the next day I will go to Our Lady of Lourdes Medical Center for a biopsy, and that I will call when it's over. No need for them to have to come, I'm sure it is nothing! Somehow, I can tell I'm not very convincing, but I pretend to play the "it's nothing" game.

This is the fourth trip to the hospital. By this time, I know the routine. I was hoping they could use my mediport instead of having to start an IV, but no such luck. The mediport was on the left and my biopsy (and possible mastectomy) was on the same side. So, start an IV, put on a hospital designer gown, and make sure that turban is on my head.

Not long afterwards my parents arrive, two close friends, and, of course, my sister Robin is there. We all joke and laugh until they come to get me. I can pretend no more. Reality is here. I swallow and begin to cry and say, "I'm scared! I don't want to do this!" Everyone in the room is trying to be strong, but everyone is crying. "We're here to support you in whatever they find," is all I can hear my Mom saying.

This time when I wake up in recovery, Sister Vernola is standing next to my bed smiling. I focus, then reach for a drain bag. There is none - halleluiah! (I'm still sedated so I don't think about checking for a breast, just a bag). Sister tells me that my family is all smiles - this one was good news. All the prayers have been answered. God is watching over me.

That night I call Toni to talk to her and I realize she has no clue as to what I have just experienced. She is concerned, but doesn't understand the severity of breast cancer. Oh well! She is only sixteen. It's better that way.

I continue to take chemo and it gets a little worse each time. It takes me longer to come out of it. I'm spending more time in bed and am still dragging when I go to work on Mondays. I don't have much sick leave left and can't afford to take leave without pay, so I must endure. It's now the end of October and I finally finish my eight and last treatment. Halleluiah.

Not much of a break. Three weeks later I am beginning six weeks of radiation. I would just start to feel better and it was time for another chemo treatment. I'm just getting better again and it is time to start radiation. Why won't they leave me alone!

It was the first part of December and the doctors told me they thought I was a candidate for a stem cell transplant. I got really angry. I can remember telling them that I had been positive through six months of chemo and now radiation. I didn't want to hear about anything medical.

For the next week or so that is all I could think about. After questioning my radiation oncologist, Dr. Deland suggested that I just go and talk to the doctors. Just because I go and ask questions doesn't mean that I am agreeing to the procedure. That sounds reasonable. As I continue radiation I continue to question the procedure. I finally agree and then am told a true shocker.

"Since you are a single parent, I suggest you get your business in order before you go to M. D. Anderson Cancer Center. There is a 10 percent chance you will come back in a box."

After several questions I was informed that most medical procedures were done with less than a one percent fatality rate. Jesus - what next!

After the initial shock I gather my wits and do as I always do - make lists of the many things that must be done. At the top of this list are a will, a living will, investments (I teach school, not many of these), credit cards and how to cancel each one, and funeral arrangements. Needless to say the two hardest were the will and funeral arrangements. It's like I am really planning to die. No. I must look at it another way. I cannot burden my only child with these decisions. Hopefully, she will not need to open those folders. However, if necessary, it would be a little easier on her.

Toni arrives the Friday before Christmas. She is exhausted. A group of her friends had a slumber party the night before; she struggled to stay awake at school; then drove to Lafayette. She is sleeping on the sofa. I let her sleep for an hour or so, then start supper. She awakens. It's at this point I tell her that we have to talk. There is business we need to discuss.

I have always been a very straightforward person, and I see no need to pad the truth now. I must tell her what to expect. I begin by saying it may be necessary for me to go to M. D. Anderson for a few months. My cancer is more serious than previously thought. I openly discuss that I will lose the hair on my head (I now have a peach fuzz of which I am quite proud), my eyebrows and eyelashes. I begin to choke when I explain that this new chemo is so strong that I may loose fingernails and toenails. When she comes to visit me it may be necessary for her to enter my room with a surgical mask, nurse's scrub, and a cap. At that point she and I are both crying. The reality is there - her mom is really sick. She had no idea that it was that bad. I then told her, "The only reason I am even agreeing to even be tested for this procedure is because of you. I love you and I want to see you grow up". We hold hands and cry. There is a long silence and she says, "I love you, Mom". Then we hug and cry more.

Later that night my ex-husband calls to speak to Toni. She is sleeping and he said not to wake her up. At that point I ask if he has a minute. I need to talk to him. It's been nine years since the divorce and I've never before asked to talk to him. I think he's shocked. I explain the situation and the possibility that I will be in Houston for several months. By this time I am crying and ask if he will give Toni permission to miss school to come to see me in Houston. My brothers have already said if he will get her to Lafayette, they would drive her to the hospital every few weeks. After all, she is the only reason I am even agreeing to this procedure. I must live a few years longer. I really didn't know how he would respond, but for the first time in nine years, he was very sympathetic. He said, "Don't worry about that - no problem. I will see that someone drives her to Lafayette and is there to pick her up on Sundays". One thing I must explain, Toni is really enjoying being a teenager. She is capable of

17

skipping school on her own. We both knew that. She has done it several times already. It will be unusual for her to miss school with permission!

I've told Toni. Now I must tell my parents. Without warning I arrive at their house Saturday morning before eight o'clock. They are drinking coffee, we share small talk, then I again say those words they dread, "I need to talk to ya'll. Something has occurred that we need to discuss." I pick my words carefully, but I must prepare them. Like Toni, I tell them what to expect. But I withhold from my parents and my daughter that there is a 10% chance I will return in a coffin. They don't need to know this.

Christmas was strained, but at least everything was out in the open. Next is New Year's Eve. Remember that celebration I was planning? Forget it. I don't feel like celebrating now, maybe next year.

January 2nd arrives. Robin and I drive to Houston, I have made arrangements to stay with a former college roommate, Susie, and she will drive us to M. D. Anderson. We arrive at her home in The Woodlands safe and sound.

The next morning very early Susie, Robin, and I take off for M. D. Anderson. It takes us over an hour in heavy traffic (now I know why I live in the country). I remember when I registered the receptionist asked for $500. After walking away I laughed and said I had met my deductible early that year. This is one of the most exhausting days I have ever lived. It took thirteen (13) hours for me to complete the preliminary tests: chest X-ray, CAT scan, bone scan, and blood work. When it was over I could hardly talk, completely exhausted. An appointment was made for me to see the doctor the next day at 2 P.M.

We got to Susie's and finally began to unwind. The phone kept ringing. It was Toni and my friends, Lou Patin and Elizabeth Fontenot. Toni really didn't understand all of this but was certainly aware that her Mom was not well. On the other hand, Lou and Elizabeth totally understood and were calling to see how I was doing - how I was holding up. I remember the stress and anxiety I felt. I hate all of this uncertainty.

January 4th - another D-Day! Susie takes Robin and me to brunch at one of the clubhouses at The Woodlands. We get in the car and Susie begins the long drive. All of a sudden there is no conversation, just silence. Everyone is stressing!

While sitting in the waiting room I really noticed the "green tint" look so many of us have - it's one of the characteristics of chemo. I am wearing a cranial prosthesis, others have very cute scarves, and others have all kinds of hats. It's amazing what a woman can do! Now they call my name. My heart is pounding. We all go to a patient room and wait. The doctor has been called to an emergency. He will be a few minutes late. What next?

After what seemed like hours, yet I was told it was only about 30 minutes, he walks into the room. My heart is about to come out of my chest. It is beating so fast. At that point I am told that after studying all the tests and conferring with other staff members, it is felt that I <u>am</u> <u>not</u> a candidate for a stem cell transplant. I am cancer free and the risk is too great. I remember thanking him for his expertise (and for rejecting me), but there was one question I had to ask.

"In your professional opinion, how much time do I have before my cancer recurs? I know that after having thirteen positive lymph nodes the likelihood of it reoccurring is high. I am being realistic. I'm the kind of person that likes to know the truth. Please be honest!"

He looked at me and took a deep breath and picked his words carefully. "I am not God, so therefore I do not have the answers to these questions. However, if I had to guess, I would say six to eight years. But remember, if you go past eight you are not cured. It takes twenty years to be cured of breast cancer." After he left the room Susie, Robin, and I just hugged each other. I was crying and couldn't stop. I remember saying, "It's over. It's finally over. No more treatments!"

In the waiting room I see a pay phone and stop to call Lou. I had promised I would call the minute I had an answer. She gets on the phone and I am crying. She asks, "Well. What did he say?" "Lou, they are not going to do it. I'm cancer free!" "Why are you crying so hard?" she asks. "Lou, I can finally rest. It's over. No more chemo treatments, no more radiation. I can finally heal. Please call my parents and Elizabeth and let them know of the decision. I'm sure they are on pins and needles." We talk for a few minutes and hang up. All of a sudden I feel as though a heavy burden has been lifted. No more indecision. That drive back to Lafayette was wonderful! I even let Robin smoke in my car. Gosh, a cigarette would be nice now, but I know I can never do that again. The doctor told me that if I started smoking again I was signing my own death certificate. The most likely place for my cancer to recur would be bones, lung, and liver.

It was April of that year that I decided to take off my cranial prosthesis. My hair was very short, but I had no bald spots, so here I go, I arrived at school (remember, I teach seventh graders) with a "Blossom" hat on my head (denim with turned up brim and a white flower). I walked into the classroom and the kids were extremely quiet. I told them that from that point on I would have short hair, but it was going to grow. I removed my hat and waited for a response. The students were real troopers. No one made fun of me. No one was mean or made a derogatory comment.

One young man who was repeating my class said, "You look ten years younger with short hair." I laughed and quickly responded, "I can assure you, making comments like that will get you everywhere. You're not going to fail!" Everyone laughed. I repeated this process of taking off my hat each hour and each time the students kept showing respect and manners. One young lady came up to me and said, "It takes a lot of courage for you to do that in front of us. I admire you." These kids are wonderful. God knew where to put me so I would receive the necessary support.

That spring I was working in my yard and my breast prosthesis was sticking to my wet skin. It was most uncomfortable. Each time I cut grass or weeded flowers beds the same thing happened. I felt miserable. So, I went to see Dr. Louis Mes, a plastic surgeon, to talk about reconstruction. At first I thought about the tram flap method, which uses your own fat but decided on saline implants (silicone implants are no longer used). Dr. Blanchet agreed with me that I might want to consider a subcutaneous mastectomy on the left breast (scoop it out) and get two implants. Remember, I had the right breast removed and a biopsy on the left one. This way I can eliminate breast cancer in my life. That's what I did - a true boob job. For the first time in my life I was going to graduate from a training bra to an adult size.

My idea of eliminating breast cancer was wrong! The following year I developed what I thought was a defect in my implants. I was going for my oncology check up, mentioned it, and asked Dr. Blanchet to check it. She does, and then says, "This is not a defect in an implant. It's a lump in your breast. Today is Monday. I would like for it to be taken care of before Friday. Please ask the surgeon to fax the results to me." My face dropped. How can this be happening? I have no breast. Oh S---!

I called Dr. Mes' office, my plastic surgeon, and made an appointment. I spoke to his nurse, told her of the lump, and that it would have to be removed. My only question was what time did they want me in the office. Did they prefer for me to be there at 7:30 A.M. or 11:30 A.M.? I wanted it removed that day. It was decided on 11:30 A.M.

This time I tell no family member, only Beth Harris, my oncology nurse. My parents can't take another scare. I arrive at the office, am prepped for the surgery, and wait for Dr. Mes to finish seeing patients. The nurses had volunteered to stay late and Dr. Mes comes into the room. He quickly removes the lump. It is completely encapsulated with clear liquid inside. It's about the size of the fingernail on my little finger. Immediately he said it was nothing to worry about, but he would have to send it to pathology to make sure. It gave me some relief that he was so confident, but I had to wait until Monday morning for the final results. When it was over, Beth smiled and winked. It appears this is only another scare. God is testing me, again.

That Friday night was the America Cancer Society fundraiser Dusk to Dawn. I stayed up all night, slept most of the day Saturday, went to bed early Saturday night, and only had to worry Sunday. That was a **long** day. Early Monday morning I call for the results of the biopsy and am given the good news. At the top of the report reads absolutely no malignancy found, no relation to breast cancer. Those words are music to my ears. It's been two years since the original diagnosis (April `93 to May `95) and I am still cancer free after two more biopsies. God is really looking after me.

March 1996 I am tutoring after school one day and my stomach begins to cramp. This continues for about half an hour; then I begin to feel as though I am having a period. Can't be! I went through menopause while taking chemo - I started menopause with my second treatment. I had a very light menstrual flow, and decided to call my oncologist. She pretended not to be alarmed but suggested I make an appointment with my gynecologist. I call and explain to the receptionist what is happening. She puts me on hold for a minute, then comes back and asks if I can go to the office the next day. Sure, I'll take off work one afternoon.

I arrive at the office, vital signs are taken, and I am put in a room and wait for the doctor to come for our pre-conference. I explain what is happening. He looks at me and says, "One of the side effects of tamoxifen is cervical cancer. I will need to do an endometrium biopsy." My facial expression must have changed dramatically because the next thing he does is ask if I am all right. I remember saying, "I don't know!"

The worst part of this procedure was waiting two days for the results. I came home from the doctor's office and checked my "cranial prosthesis" - I may need it again. My colleagues at work commented that I looked tired and drained, but I denied that anything was wrong. I had told no family members about this. I can't let it slip now. When I did get the results everything was negative. Oh God, you have answered my prayers. Thanks for listening and agreeing with me, again.

Everything goes well and two years later the same thing happens - I start spotting. I just called the doctor, explained the situation, and asked if he wanted to do an endometrium biopsy, again. For some reason I am just a little afraid, and I am beginning to wonder when my luck will run out. One of these days something will be malignant - just don't let it be today! My Dad is in the hospital because of complications from a stroke he had several years before. My parents can't deal with me getting sick again now. It's Friday and the nurses say they can't give me results. Only the doctor can do that. Between classes I use the phone and he is always with a patient. Finally, I am in tears and stressing to the max. It's time for me to go to the hospital and I know I can't call from there. I know I can't wait until Monday. By this time I am crying on the phone and the doctor speaks to me between patients. "Everything is OK, don't worry," he says. Again the burden is lifted. Again I beat the odds. Five biopsies and only the first one was malignant. A friend of mine says, "God isn't finished with you, yet. He's keeping you on earth for a reason." Time will only tell the reason, I've learned not to question.

The summers of `98 and `99 also had a surprise for me. In June of both years, I had to have skin cancers removed from my back. The dermatologists said they were the result of too much sun exposure as a child. Both times just the simple surgery in his office sufficed. Again God is taking care of me.

Up to this point I have discussed only the depressing side of cancer. I felt this was necessary in hopes of giving someone else an opportunity to see what I had been through and they would know that they, too, can live through five biopsies. I feel there are two other phases I need to discuss: the good thing that resulted from my being diagnosed and the funny things that happened to me. Anyone who knows me knows that I fought this disease using a lot of humor. Hell, you either cry or laugh and I prefer to laugh. As you have read, I did cry a lot and I feel that was part of the healing process. But I also laughed a lot and that was the best medicine. Earlier, I mentioned that my daughter was 16 years old when I was diagnosed. She had chosen to go and live with her dad at age 13, returned to me, and had gone back to his home. The second time it was understood there was no coming back permanently - the musical house game was over. Needless to say our relationship was strained. After being diagnosed we realized we did not have time to waste. Instead of arguing when we disagreed, one of us would say, "This conversation is not going well. I think it is best if we stop and talk about it later". That was a sign to layoff or it was going to explode. Why didn't we do this years ago? Life would have been so much easier.

Several of us met regularly at the oncologist's office, we received chemo on the same schedule. After chemo we missed each other. We would get on the phone and check with one another regularly. Beth Harris formed the Our Lady Of Lourdes Breast Cancer Survivors. I have been active in this group for over six years. The old faithfuls still show up occasionally, but this old faithful goes regularly. Elizabeth Geubler Ross once said there was a sixth stage of grief - reaching out and helping others. I have found this stage most rewarding. I got to know other women who have been diagnosed, help to answer their questions and lessen their fears. When I do this I feel a wonderful sense of accomplishment. With 13 positive lymph nodes, I would like to think I give them lots of hope and encouragement. Dr. Mes once showed us an article in a medical magazine that said there was a tendency to believe that women who belong to a support group live longer than those that do not belong to one. Stop and think. I don't want to be the one that does not show up for the next meeting because of medical reasons, would you?

Several times friends have approached me and said that a friend of theirs was diagnosed with cancer and they wanted to know what they could do to help. My first response is prayer and my second is food. In one way I was fortunate because I was by myself and did not have to feel responsible for others (food, clean clothes, chauffeuring kids, etc.) If you really want to help someone, prepare a meal for the family. Personally, I couldn't move my right arm for three weeks. I don't know how I could have stirred a pot, much less prepared a meal. The faculty members of Judice Middle School fed me for six weeks. During that time a hot meal was brought to my home seven days a week for six weeks. If it hadn't been for them life would have been a lot more difficult. To each I will be forever grateful. To this day I keep them in my prayers.

Before it was allowed, my co-workers at JMS had planned to donate two weeks sick leave to me. This would assure that when I went on Sabbatical Leave, I would not be docked two weeks leave on a paycheck. This was called "The Twelve Days of Christmas for Martha." When Elizabeth went to ask faculty members with a lot of accumulated sick leave to help, she was amazed at the response. Before she knew it, over a month was being donated. The principal, Robert Adamson, told me he would do it as long as he didn't get caught. (He was already of retirement age, very well respected in education circles, and had nothing to lose.) I was to prepare lesson plans for two weeks. A substitute teacher would be placed in my room and one of my co-workers would fill out the paperwork for sick leave. This was a true gift from the heart. Because the stem cell transplant was not necessary, this sick leave was never needed. However, their kindness will never be forgotten. (Now, sick leave can be donated. In 1993 this was not approved.)

When telling people my story I like to include my favorite rejection in my life - M. D. Anderson. I say that I have experienced divorce and my child moving out of my house twice. But, being turned down from that stem cell transplant was great. "I have never been so happy to be a reject!"

If anyone has ever been faced with an extended illness, you know that there are many household chores that must be taken care of, one of which is the yard. That old grass will continue to grow and I have to find someone to take care of this chore. My neighbor's son, Brandt, was in sixth grade. I asked his parents if I could hire him to cut grass once a week and asked what they thought would be adequate compensation. His dad looked at me and said, "He has to learn to do things for people in need and not to always be paid for his efforts. He will do it for free!" My medical expenses were about to skyrocket. I couldn't believe what I was hearing. Yet, I felt he deserved some compensation. We agreed that I would take him to the restaurant of his choice and let him order whatever he wanted. We did this about every two weeks. I was amazed at the amount of fried chicken, tacos, French fries, malts, etc. that a boy could consume. I laughed with his mom and told her I probably would have come out cheaper paying him. (Not true, but a good joke).

I mentioned two very good friends that over the years have seen me through thick and thin. Life had thrown me a few curves and they had always been there to help me. I truly believe that we have many acquaintances in life, but only a few true friends. Lou Patin and Elizabeth Fontenot are true friends.

I'll begin with Lou. We met about fifteen years ago and hit it off immediately. Many people that meet her are intimidated by her strong will personality, yet I never saw her in that light. She is a very determined person that sets goals and achieves them. She is the only person I know that could go into the employment agency business when Lafayette was facing a recession and be in the black within a year. That's determination. I have always admired that quality in her.

We both get involved in our work and family life and may go weeks without talking to each other. Yet, when one of us needs the other, we just call and support is there immediately. Lou was with me through all stages of my ordeal. She came to see me in the hospital, brought food to my home, and spent time with me cheering me up. She would call and do anything I asked of her.

I found out after the fact that when I was going for my second breast biopsy, Lou was very concerned about my health and about my daughter. She could see that Toni had no idea of what I was experiencing, nor did Toni realize the severity of my disease. I found out later that Lou had decided if that second lump had been malignant, she was going to drive two hours to meet my ex-husband and talk to my daughter. She was going to make Toni realize that my time on this earth may be limited. She had planned to encourage her to come to Lafayette, at least every other weekend. I had expressed to Lou many times, that if it weren't for Toni, I would quit chemo and let the chips fall. However, I needed to see her grow up. She was constantly encouraging me to go on, that I had a lot of life left in me. When I was depressed she would come to get me out of the house.

Lou has seen me with hair, with no hair, with no breast, and with fake ones. She has helped me to laugh through all of this. She is a true friend.

Elizabeth is the other true friend that has helped me through many bad times. By the time I was diagnosed in 1993 we had worked together for seven years and had become very close. She and Lou had both helped me through a divorce and my daughter going to live with her dad, returning to me then going back. Now it was cancer and they both stuck with me again.

Elizabeth was the one that organized the "Feed Martha Campaign." A hot meal was delivered to my house seven days a week for six weeks. Monday through Friday, the teachers would bring the meal to school and Elizabeth would deliver it and stay with me for a few hours. She would always cheer me up, no matter how down I had become.

I remember one day I was crying. I was so depressed. The last time I had hit such a low point in life I was going through my only child leaving home. Elizabeth walked in the back room; I thought she had gone to the bathroom. She reappeared in my den, pretending to be a two hundred pound woman (she only weights 110 pounds). She had every pillow in my house in her shirt and skirt. As she walked they fell. I started laughing so hard I was crying. She looked at me and said, "It worked, you're no longer crying". I found out a year later that she would go home and cry. Her husband had to console her.

January 1998 is another example that out of everything bad comes something good. I was one of ten breast cancer survivors from throughout the United States selected to appear on the Rosie O'Donnell Show. Elizabeth and I flew to New York, walked Broadway until midnight and were picked up the next morning in a limo and taken to the studio. We were walking down a hall and were taken to a dressing room. Once inside I looked at her and said, "That's the hall they show on "Saturday Night Live," the one with pictures of all the guest hosts." We then made an excuse to go to the bathroom so we could see the pictures again.

A young man came to the dressing room to bring me a script to follow to introduce the show. I practiced it a few times, then, we went to the studio. I practiced once or twice with the teleprompter and then it was time for all the guests to be seated in the studio. A comedian entertained us, got us pumped up, and then it was time for the show.

Before getting out of my seat, Elizabeth and I were talking and laughing. I remember telling her, "I'm going to have a good time. I'm also going to make my family proud of me. And, most of all, I want Louisiana to have a good image. I'm so tired of all the negative publicity we have gotten lately." I took a deep breath, smiled, and introduced the show. Rosie came out and we joked for a long time. We were going "Tit - for - tat". It was wonderful.

That appearance afforded me the opportunity to speak at several functions in the Lafayette area - to give other breast cancer survivors hope. That's what reaching out and helping others is all about.

One of my greatest assets is my ability to laugh at this disease and myself. I would like to share some of the funny things that happened. I had to go to see an urologist and his nurse came in the room to check blood pressure, etc. Then she said, "Who does your hair? I love it! I have been trying to find someone to cut my hair just like that!" I looked at her and laughed. "Lady, you don't understand! This is bought. I'm on chemo and am bald." She was so embarrassed, and began to apologize. I laughed and thanked her for the compliment.

The America Heart Association had a Monte Carlo night and I went with Lou because her husband did not want to go. Well, they are giving away door prizes. Guess what I won? It was a free haircut and style from a local boutique. Lou begins cackling and letting everyone know that I am wearing a wig because I have no hair on my head.

Just prior to going to M. D. Anderson I am organizing all my business affairs. I tell Elizabeth that I have everything in order, but am including a hand written note with my will. I want close personal friends and family members to have certain mementos. I'm really on my "pity-pot." She looks at me, just as serious as can be, and said, "You know that lamp you have behind your sofa?" I started laughing and said, "You Bitch." "It got you to laugh, again."

One summer I went hiking in the Santa Fe and Sandia Mountains in New Mexico. While there I noticed my left breast slowly deflating. When I returned to Lafayette I went to see my plastic surgeon. He laughed and called it a "flat tire." So, here I go again - another surgery. I told him that if it was necessary for me to go through all that pain again, I just as well get larger implants. He agreed. I got a size larger, and for someone who has always been very flat chested, this is great!

There are days that I still feel sorry for myself like the day I was talking to Elizabeth Fontenot. I'm telling her that one day I may want to remarry, how could a man look at me, I only had one breast. Very seriously she responds, "Tell him to get drunk and cross his eyes. He'll see two." I just looked at her and laughed.

Cancer has taught me another of life's lessons, I will never have another "bad hair" day. I've got hair and that makes it a good day!

I hope I have given cancer patients and their families an insight into this journey and the realization that you too can face obstacles and overcome them. Remember my favorite quote: "The greatest thing in this world is not so much where we are, but in what direction we are moving."

Think positive. Move forward. Embrace life.

Neppie's Story

I was not what you would call a happy child. My first recollection was during Hurricane Audrey in 1957. I was told that this was one of the most disastrous storms in History. No wonder I remember it so vividly. I can remember holding my favorite doll's hand. You know the one we all had to have in the 50's. She was five feet tall, looked like a real little girl, and was supposed to be able to wear our own clothes. There was only one problem with my doll and me. My clothes were entirely too big for my doll. You see I was a chubby little girl.

My Maw Maw kept telling me not to go outside but I was too curious and probably a little defiant. So I went out anyway. She lived in a middle-class subdivision. It was wonderful there and every time she came to visit my mom and dad I packed my little red suitcase and dropped it by the door. That meant that I was going home with her and my Pa Pa. This visit was exciting to me and scary to everyone else. I was too little to know that we were in danger. I escaped out the side screen door with my favorite doll and then it happened.

The force of the wind picked that doll and me up and threw us into the neighbor's yard. It all happened within seconds but at that moment I was aware that something bigger than me was in the universe. I was scared. Actually, I have been scared most of my life. I have never trusted adults. They were supposed to make my life safe. They made my life hell. I always felt like a burden and always felt like I was in the way. I picked up the weight of the world at age six and I tried desperately to carry it. I was a wreck. I slept too much and ate too much. These things gave me pleasure. This was the only time that I had peace and it was something that I could enjoy. I was paralyzed with fear. My parents fought. They fought over each other, fought over my sister and me, fought over money and over nothing. It didn't matter what it was, they just liked to fight or so it seemed to a six-year-old girl. I learned to hate conflict. To me it meant pain and hurt all of the time. I had no peace when they were around. I felt no love. A child must feel loved or they die a little each day. It is so sad to be a child in a hostile environment. My mother did the best she could when they divorced; but it was not popular in those days to be divorced. We moved to another city, New Orleans. The dreaded New Orleans Projects was our home. There were some very colorful neighbors who lived there. For some reason I blocked most of them out of my memory; but there were drunks, peeping Toms, and a lady who lived around us with real long hair and we actually thought that she was a witch. She sure scared a lot of little kids and I was one. It wasn't safe there but that was our home. We did the best we could and always made good grades so mom would be proud of us. I took care of my sister Jessica and we survived.

My life changed about age nine when my mother remarried and my stepfather took us to North Louisiana to live. We had a new family and they were safe. There was no more fighting and fussing and there were lots of family activities. Things were good until I became a teenager.

Why am I so unhappy? I'm always trying to get attention, especially from the opposite sex. They all say I'm pretty. I diet to excess and become thin but I never feel thin enough. Why is it so important to me that I please boys and why does it make me feel so empty? I'm very popular but I never feel happy. Who am I? I cry and I cry. It seems I've spent my whole life crying. When I was older my Maw Maw told me a story about how I used to cry all of the time and she told me that if I did not stop crying so much my eyes would fall out. Well, every morning all of us would stumble to the breakfast table and were presented with coffee milk, a tradition in Cajun households. I drank my coffee milk and as I took the last swallow I almost choked when two big green eyes were looking back at me from the bottom of that glass. I started rubbing my eyes cause I knew she was right and my eyes finally fell out from crying too much. I think that must have been the day I decided not to cry and to hold in all of those emotions from then on. Big Mistake!!

I survived my teenage years and graduated from high school, entered Northeast College in Monroe at the age of 16. In my sophomore year, I transferred to the University of Southwestern Louisiana and I made Lafayette, Louisiana, my home. I married, had three beautiful daughters in four years and I thought life was good. I loved being a mom. The marriage lasted 15 years but there was lots of sadness and mental abuse. The divorce was bitter but I was determined that I would work as many jobs as I needed to provide a home for my girls. We cried a lot and ate a lot of tuna fish and salads but we survived. My husband told me that no other man would want me with three kids. Wrong! One of his friends was waiting to pick up the pieces. I don't know if I was just scared or flattered or both but I started seeing him. It made me feel better and he took me places. However, I didn't have time to heal. You need that time to find out who you are. I married "Tom" and it was a struggle from the beginning.

I had to always be the person he wanted to be proud of. I was made to feel like I could never go out in public unless I was perfectly dressed (what he considered perfect) low cut dresses or blouses, short skirts, heels, and makeup. I tried my best to please him and it only caused me pain. I exercised excessively, didn't eat much because he didn't like fat. My life was Hell and I felt trapped. I didn't want another divorce. I died a little each day and I tried to please even more. I was becoming an imposter.

Exercise has always taken stress away from my life and I was diagnosed at age 10 with scoliosis so exercise was a very important part of my daily routine. In 1996, I started feeling fatigued and turned to a friend who is a personal trainer. She had just opened her own business and I joined her exercise program. My body started taking on a beautiful new shape and I was proud. My husband was proud too. However, I was pushing myself to attend class. I liked the way I looked but it was exhausting. I kept telling myself that it was the price I had to pay for looking good in my clothes and it would go away. It was on one of those exercise days that I felt something suspicious in my chest. As I did a series of arm curls, I felt pain. I reached into my blouse and felt a thickening, not a lump but almost like a keloid scar. I dismissed it as part of my chest enhancement from the exercise but I could not keep my hands off that spot. My gynecologist, during a routine exam, had found what she thought might be something. I have fibrocystic breasts and, since I had never had a mammogram, she suggested that we get a base mammogram to be on the safe side. I put it in my purse and forgot about it until I felt that thickening. I didn't know what it was. I came home and jumped in the shower. My daughter, Shannon, came into the bathroom to ask me a question. I asked her to feel the thickening. She said, "Mom, I don't know what that is but whatever it is, it doesn't belong there." That's all I kept hearing during the night in my head was "it doesn't belong there." Now, I was scared. Tomorrow I will deal with this, not today, but tomorrow.

I pulled the mammogram order out of my purse and I called the Women and Children's Hospital for an appointment. Surely they would tell me that this was okay. The nurse asked me where the spot was that I was worried about. I showed her and she marked it with a black magic marker. Now I was scared. I stood there bare-chested and they told me the doctor would like to talk to me. He barged into the room and said, "How long has this been there? This is cancer and we need to get you into surgery today." He addressed the nurse and asked if we could do this at 1:00. I guess the look on my face told him that I was not going to do this today and he basically attacked me. He said, "You want me to call your doctor? He will tell you the same thing." Not only did the doctor get my name wrong, he was irate that I would not let him do the biopsy. I went to my gynecologist's office at 1:00 p.m. She said, "I agree that it does look like cancer and we need to talk to a surgeon, but let's talk about living." That was the first ray of hope that I found. She called and arranged an appointment with a surgeon on the next day. He agreed that it looked like cancer but we would have to go in to make sure. We scheduled the surgery in a few days and at that time I would have to make decisions. If it were cancer, my doctor would need to know what to do at that time. I couldn't make the word mastectomy come out. Cancer was something that old people got, not women in their 40's. I thought all people died that had cancer. I felt numb. I could not think. I didn't even have a clue about what questions to ask. I just thought I was going to die!

After I found out that I had to have surgery, "Tom" took me to the grocery store. I picked up ice cream, chocolate covered peanuts, M & M's, and potato chips. He said, "Nep, what are you doing?" I said, "If I'm gonna die, I want to taste these things again." I have been good. I have been eating salads, broccoli, apples, and orange juice. Why did this happen? We turned the corner and started down another aisle. I came face to face with Connie and Gerald from work. Connie has the heart of a saint and hugged me. "We're all proud of you, you're giving the rest of us courage." Why did she have to say that? Now I knew I wouldn't eat all of those snacks. I would have courage. I want to **live**.

I wasn't scared at that point. I just wanted to enjoy some of the "good things" in life. I was concerned that everyone would have enough food while I was sick. Instead, they all fed me when I was recovering. I was so thankful and so was my family. I'll never forget the day Ms. Lil came with a roast, green beans, a homemade lemon meringue pie, and a beautiful flower from her garden. I felt so loved. We all love Mrs. Lil, and her beautiful spirit, and of course, I was so thankful my children ate so good that day.

I wanted to cry. I wanted to scream. God, this was so unfair. We all go to the hospital. My sister Jessica comes in town and my friend Dana comes all the way from Florida just to be there with me. We laughed in the waiting room and acted like it would be okay. I was so scared. A friend of my husband was there. His wife was having surgery. She has been suffering for a long time. The surgeon came out quickly, "I'm sorry your wife has liver cancer and there is nothing that we can do. She will have about three months to live." She was only a few years older than me. Great. That was not what I needed to hear right before they took me into surgery. "Please God," I prayed, "Let me be okay. I want to live. I'm not prepared to die. I want to see my granddaughter, Hailey grow up."

They call my name. I wish that I could disappear. My family hugs me like I will not see them again. We go into the back and they ask me to undress and put that beautiful gown on. Bobby, the anesthesiologist and friend, comes in and starts the procedure to put me to sleep. Some of my friends who are nurses in the operating room come over talk to me and it gives me courage to know that they are around. One of the nurses comes in to say hello, and tells me that she lived across the street from me when I was five years old. I wish someone could take my place. "Why me?"

I feel dizzy. "Neppie, Neppie. Wake up." I try but I am too sleepy. I ask what time it is? And I am told it is 1:00 pm. It's been too long. I know this in my heart. My thoughts in my head begin to whirl around like the sound of a washer. I knew it must be cancer. Then the nurse whispers, "You had a mastectomy." It's over. I close my eyes but I have to disagree, it's not over. This is just the beginning. I sleep.

Why are you screaming at me? Mom, Mom, wake up. I'm here. I made it Mom. It's Shawn, my daughter. I start to cry. I try to wake up —-why is it so hard? Why do I hurt so much? What happened? Oh God, no. It's true, mastectomy. I see a porcelain angel in a flower arrangement that my friend Laura sent to me and I realize where I am. I pray that I am not dying. There are so many people in this room. I have lots of friends and family. I go back to sleep. There is not much to say. My Aunt Linda and Uncle John come to visit me. I cry and tell Uncle John that I was not prepared to die. I do not have a will. I do not have a cemetery plot. I cannot afford to die right now. Not today, not tomorrow. Uncle John, in his absolutely wonderful humor, says I can be buried with him and Aunt Linda, only if we promise to bury him in the middle of us two…and of course, the laughter came and this helped me to come back to my reality, my reality of today. I knew in my heart he was serious, and I then am able to relax. They both love me so much. My sister, Jessica, stays with me and I must look bad because she asks if I'm gonna throw up. I don't realize I am but here it comes. I hate to throw up but projectile vomiting is different. (I hate carrots to this day. They remind me of that day.) About 2 a.m. I call the nurse who happens to be a guy and ask for a Sprite. He brings it to me and I ask for a straw. "Okay, he said, "I'll bring it to you but straws give you gas!" I burst out laughing. "Lord, please, I am strong but I can't handle the loss of my breast and gas both on the same day." To this day I still cannot drink out of a straw without thinking about the nurse and that gas! At least I knew I could laugh. I hadn't lost my sense of humor. I cannot sleep, so I walk up and down the hall. The nurses look startled when they see me. I almost trip over a statue of the Virgin Mary, and for some Catholic reason, I fall to my knees, and begin to cry. I am scared, really scared, and feel very alone. I say a little prayer and sit next to that statue for a while then I feel a peace, stop crying, and I know I'll be okay.

Dr. Carroll has me stay another day. My youngest daughter, Shelly, stays with me. She is studying to become a nurse and the nurses call her "Little Bit." They train her to empty my drains and clean the dressing, measure and document everything. I am so scared. She learns quickly and I feel proud and lucky to have such wonderful care. We go home. I won't look at the bandage. I never look down. I avoid all mirrors. I want this all to go away. The cancer part has not even hit me yet. I am still grieving the loss of the breast.

At first my husband seemed supportive but my grieving would last too long for him. Slowly he would distance himself.

The reports were in. The cancer had not spread. We picked an oncologist and made an appointment. I was concerned with things like percentages, side effects, and life expectancy. My husband could only ask about reconstruction. Dr. Brierre, my oncologist, frowned. The trouble began. That is when I truly faced the reality that I was defective to him.

One day I would feel on top of the world and the next day I thought God had called my number. That's the way you feel on chemo. Don't let me say everyone. Everyone does not feel the same way. My first visit to the oncologist was a story in itself. The building was cold, no not cold, freezing. It was June and now I had stopped feeling sorry for myself. I was wearing my sleeveless t-shirts and summer appropriate clothing again. But now I was freezing, I wondered what I would see in that office. I really didn't have a clue. No one can prepare you for such an experience. Why would anyone talk about chemo if they didn't have to? I entered the room and there were old people there that day and they all looked real sick. I didn't want to look like them and I got scared. Oprah was on T.V. and no one looked at each other. Some had hair. Some had wigs. Some had scarves or hats. It was obvious to everyone there that I either had finished my chemo a long time ago or I hadn't even started. Would I look like these people? It had been 30 days and I felt human again.

Now what? I can remember there was a door from the waiting room where the nurse would call you. It was locked and there was a button they had to push to let you in. Did they really think that any of us would just rush past that door to get injected with our medicine? I shook inside. There were signs all over saying please do not wear perfume or body lotions in consideration of chemo patients. What did that mean? I soon found out! The smell of perfume caused projectile vomiting...for me.

Dr. Brierre said we had to do four chemo sessions and we would try to do them in my right arm with one nurse. It would be slow and would take longer for my visits but I wouldn't have to have the mediport surgery. I don't like the word surgery and I jumped on that idea. Thank God there was one good thing going my way. The nurse looked at my veins and shook her head. Nurses have done that all of my life. Tiny veins. We tried. She came and asked me to sit in a chair especially for chemo recipients. It was a padded chair with a stiff-arm rest. Some people looked sick, kind of a grayish color, no hair, little sprigs of hair, wigs (it was obvious), and then there was me, the newest member of their sorority. Damn, I hate these sorority things, especially this one. You had two choices, die or live. I chose the latter. She took a blood sample to test and see if I was healthy. I passed the first test. I had been resting, a lot, and eating really healthy. Isn't that the way it is? You have an aversion to potato chips after the fact. Those beer and nachos were great but wouldn't the veggies have helped me not get in this predicament in the first place? Maybe! Maybe not! Dear God what the hell is this all about? I don't want to learn this life lesson and if it is okay with you, please give it to someone else. No dice! My number must be on this dance card. She (the nurse) comes towards me with the biggest vial of red Kool-Aid looking liquid. I kept thinking how could this be going into those little veins of mine. She tells me to take a big breath and relax. "How?" I feel like everyone is looking at me. When you look into the eyes of all those chemo patients together in one room it's a strange experience. The eyes are sad. It's like looking into their souls. There's nothing there at the moment the "medicine" is going in. You feel so powerless. You feel so vulnerable. Someone else at that moment is controlling your life. We don't know what else to do. We are thankful our number hasn't been pushed but at the same time you have to wonder if you will see any of these people again. You don't really want to become friends with them because they may not be there next week. It's hard to explain. But somewhere deep inside your soul you know that you have been with this person before or you will see them again. Somewhere. Somehow. They have touched your soul and their faces would always be engraved in your memory. Don't need to know their earthly names. They will always be a part of your being.

I'm given something to help the nausea. For that kindness, I am so thankful. Dear God, thank you, if I am worthy, please give me another chance to live. So far I've managed to make a mess of my life but I can learn. My lessons are mine and I will study and do better. Just give me that chance. You make a lot of deals with God when you think you might be close to death. You pray all of the time and you wonder why you were the <u>chosen one</u>. I sometimes think God chose us to test the people around us. Let's see who knows how to love. I was told, at my support group meeting, that I would be surprised at how people reacted to my cancer. Everyone would handle it differently and in his or her own way. After all, none of us are prepared for cancer. I didn't know how to handle cancer either. Cancer happened to old people, people I didn't know, not to women in their prime time of life. Cancer snuck up on me in the middle of the night. It stole my peace.

My doctor said to make sure I did not get pregnant. That would have been a miracle since I had my tubes tied 23 years ago and my husband had a vasectomy not to mention he found making love a duty instead of love. I always wore my bra because when I was without it he turned his face in disgust. He didn't hold me anymore. I learned not to dress or undress in front of him. I learned he didn't really love me. He needed help but he was too proud to ask for it. For our anniversary he rented the hotel room that we shared on our honeymoon. There was only one problem. It had a hot tub. I agonized over what to wear in that tub. I finally had to know if the relationship would work and I decided to do the tub in the nude. I lit candles all around and bought a CD player with the most romantic music. I slipped into the bubbles. Everything was okay until the bubbles disappeared. My heart raced, how would he react? He became extremely aware of my missing breast. He turned white and then started coughing like he was going to throw up. I knew in my heart it was over. He said I wasn't his sexy wife anymore. He couldn't accept me without a breast and I couldn't live with someone who was ashamed of me because I had lost one to cancer. I knew people loved me but he was not one of them.

You might say I was reborn on that day. I was free. It was over. Now I was able to ask God to redirect my life so I could learn what true love was all about. I wanted a good friend, a wonderful, loving, and kind person. I am here to say, be very careful what you ask for, because you just might get that and more, in a good sort of way.

It seems my angels had been looking out for me for quite some time. I have a friend in my life. His name is Freddy. He's eight years younger than I am and I have known him since he was ten. The cancer brings him back into my life. He calls Shelly to check on me, fixes things around the house, cooks, and cheers us all up. Everyone loves him and we all grow to cherish his friendship. At some point I realize that if he doesn't stop by every day I really miss him. One day Shelly, my youngest daughter, sat me down and said, "Mom, I'm not gonna let you screw this up. Freddy is too special. Don't you realize he is in love with you?" I didn't have a clue. Freddy says I wasn't paying attention. Maybe that's true but I can tell you the minute, the place, the time, and the feelings I had when I fell in love with him. My mom, dad, children, and Stella were at my home for Christmas. It was cold and sleeting. The fire was roaring, everyone was laughing, and visiting. Stella, Freddy, and I were sitting at my kitchen table. We had just given Stella her present, and she and Freddy were talking and laughing, and I became very peaceful. I felt warmth and a voice that said, "Now you are loved and now you know how to love." It's unlike anything I had ever experienced. I finally know what true love is. I knew at that moment I would be with this person for the rest of my life and my life would be beautiful.

In January around the 11th, Freddy and I went to see a movie, "Patch Adams." I cried. I guess Freddy decided it was time for "our talk". He told me that he had been in love with me for quite some time and loved my children and grandchild. He then asked me to share my life with him. His Uncle John is married to my Aunt Linda so we have mutual family. During my illness, I prayed that God would show me how love should feel between a man and a woman and that I receive a love like Aunt Linda and Uncle John's. Be careful what you ask for.

I was afraid, petrified of Freddy's reaction to my missing breast but I knew in my heart that it would make no difference. Freddy laughed and assured me he loved me as a person, as a spiritual being and not for what body parts I had or didn't have. He said, "I love you because of the person I become when I am with you and I want to be with you forever." I understood and I felt the same way. We are best friends and to me he is one of those angels on earth.

I knew in my heart that this time I would not be rejected. I'll never forget the first time he saw my scar. He said, "Oh, that's what you were worried about. Sweetheart, that's nothing. It just lets me be closer to your heart." You had to loose a breast so your heart could learn how to love. The loss of that breast allowed me to love again, I thought. I cried. One day I was looking in the mirror after my bath. He slipped his arms around my waist and told me I was beautiful. "She, my right breast, must be lonely." I said. "Oh no," he said, "She's having all the fun. Think about it. No competition!" We both started laughing and I fell into his arms, lovingly kissed him and thanked God for such a wonderful friend and partner.

The wedding was beautiful. June 2, 2000, almost four years to the day of being diagnosed with breast cancer, and one year to the day Loretta, Martha, Stella and I met to talk about starting the book. Stella always said it would be a rebirth. Wow. Over 200 of our closest friends attended our wedding. It was an old time Cajun wedding complete with horse and carriage. Our children were all in the wedding, even my granddaughter and unborn grandsons Braden Isaiah and Garret Jude. You could feel the love in that church. We made memories, memories that will stay in our hearts forever. Cancer cannot take those away. We are family and we are love. I can now love and I can now accept love; our life is so beautiful. Our shared love grew out of **our** battle with breast cancer. Freddy rallied to my side when others retreated and we fell deeply in love; our life involves everyday acts of intimacy, and affection. We respect each other and we are best friends. Best friends do not hurt each other. We laugh and we cry together…this must be what God meant when he said, "Love one another as I Love you."

The loss of a breast was a small price to pay for such a beautiful rich loving life that I now know. It took the loss of my breast for me to focus on the important things in life. I am at peace now. My heart is open. I love myself. I love my body, not for the physical appearance but for the simple reason that it was chosen to house my soul. I was pure at birth and then the world got to me. Somewhere along the way I was robbed of its innocence. How sad but after I started to remake my life, I learned from the past. I learned that I couldn't change another person, but I could find the inner strength to walk away and take care of what I know is right for me. I learned how to recognize love from lust. I learned how to give of my heart but only to those who are honest. I learned to listen to my heart and trust those who are worthy. I learned how to love and how to allow myself to be loved. It feels good. Could I have learned to love myself without going through cancer? Maybe, maybe not. I can't go backwards, I can't live in the past. I have learned from my lessons. I'm not saying that I won't make mistakes but I am saying that I am more open to the universe. I don't worry about the small stuff, the things I cannot change. Worry is a waste of energy. I am more compassionate and more loving. When I look at a child I see God. All children are born so innocent, so connected to God. It takes so little time for the world to get to them and change their little souls. How sad. Why can't we stay connected forever? Wouldn't it be a beautiful world for all of us? That's not the way it is though. We must all get through our lessons here on earth the best way we can.

At this point in my life I try to enjoy every minute. God let me live through cancer and win the battle. For that I am grateful. I try not to panic when I have a headache, a stomachache, or even a cold. It's normal for a "C" patient to panic. For the most part we have a normal life, we forget the big "C" and go on with our normal activities. But when an ache or pain creeps up we always wonder if it's back.

When I schedule maintenance tests, I become a totally different person. I am antsy and on edge or just plain scared. I can't see my insides and most of the time cancer doesn't hurt. My destiny is in the hands of the God and my physicians. I get anxiety attacks. I pray as my blood is taken and I cringe as they literally smash my breast in the mammogram machine. All of my life I have been told to be careful with my breast. Don't mash or bruise them and then I pay them to do this to me! Someone, the man who invented this machine, should have this experience. I know if a woman had invented this machine, she would have considered gravity. This can't be good for a healthy breast. The tech always comes back into the room and wants to take another picture. She sees the scar tissue from my surgery that goes into the other breast. The radiologist told the tech that she was wrong. It was just scar tissue. The tech was disturbed that she wouldn't be able to take another test and marched into the room and told me I could go. Man, she loves finding stuff in my breasts. I'm glad she's conscientious but she loves scaring me every time.

I guess I will always be a little nervous about life, my life that is. Freddy never leaves home without giving me a hug, kiss, I love you. He hugs me every night and thanks me for sharing my life and my children with him. I have to remind him that it's our life, our children, and our love. My angels, no, our angels were always around watching over us. Just waiting for both of us to pay attention! We both know one day this "C" may return. But I won't be alone this time. I will be afraid but I also will be loved and supported. The big "C" took away a breast but opened my heart so I could receive love, give love, and cherish love. My darling Freddy, we all love you. I want to live. I want to love you and share this happiness for a long time.

My girls are my life. I know God loves me tremendously because he chose me to be the instrument to bring them into this world. They have been my strength. I know that I could not have been as strong if I wasn't fighting for them. A mother will find the inner strength to protect her children. I love them more than life itself. They are so precious to me. They gave me the will to live. Hailey, Braden, and Garret, you are my grandchildren and I want to hold you in my arms, and in my heart; I want to hear "I Love You, MiMi" for a long, long time. I want to live. I want to see each of you grow up. Thank you Shawn, Shannon, and Shelly, my children, I Love You. You held my hand and watched me suffer. You, my darlings, gave me the will to fight. I cherish each day that I am allowed to remain here on earth with you. I am so proud of the beautiful, strong, loving women you have become. And Freddy, I am totally in love with you and thank you for teaching me to love myself. I will always cherish your love, and your heart, for you have taught me how to truly be alive.

Loretta's Story

Christmas 1995

Can't go exercise. It's Christmas. I'm going to Lake Charles to be with my family. Bruce has gone to be with his family. We'll be together later. Take a bath. What's this? A lump in my left breast. I tell myself not to worry. It's just one of those fibroid things I've been told I have. Now that I've lost 20 pounds and am exercising regularly I can feel it. *Don't worry, it's only been six months since your last mammogram and nothing was there. You have a mammogram every year. It's only fibroid things.*

I will just go to Lake Charles and not say anything. But knowing me, I won't be able to keep my mouth shut. I will have to tell my mother. *Don't worry; it's nothing.*

I guess I didn't worry about it. I was too happy with my life. I had a new job that I liked and I was in love. Bruce was there for me. I seemed to be important to him. We laughed together, we fished together, and we loved together. Life was good. Nothing bad could happen to me again.

January 2000

I notice how firm I am getting. Exercising as often as 5 times a week is paying off. Well, my body is firm, especially my left breast. As I look in the mirror, I like my body. It looks better than ever. Now I need to work more on the right breast to firm it up too.

February, Valentine's Day 1996

Things are going well but I feel a little tired. It's more than normal. It's just the exercise and work. Sleep late this Sunday and catch up. Bruce stays over. He gets up before me. How nice to have someone take care of you for a while. Can smell the coffee.

Wait a minute. Something's wrong. Now I'm worried. My left breast didn't look right. It almost looks like two pieces to one breast. Something is wrong. Now I'm scared. I promise to go to the doctor.

The next day, Monday, I call the doctor and make an appointment for Tuesday. Dr. Hawes, such a fatherly figure, looks at me with concern, but not to frighten me. He makes an appointment for me to see a surgeon. I meet Bruce there that afternoon.

OK, this is going to be nothing. One of those fibroid things that just got big. But why is the doctor talking this way? What is he saying? It's something about cancer. Guess I'm not listening. He's talking about someone else, not me, just general terms. Not me. Bruce, why are you looking that way? What's that? He wants to biopsy. Why does it feel different when he examines it? What is he saying? I'm not sick. I'm healthy. I eat right and get lots of exercise. Bruce, why are you looking that way? OK, doctor, I'll schedule a biopsy, outpatient. Yes, insurance will cover. What mastectomy? No! Not me, not now. Second opinion. Anyway, it's not me he's talking about. Let's just go back to work. The biopsy will show them. It'll prove there is nothing. I'm healthy.

At the office, I tell Norma, my boss. It's still not me. Nothing really made sense. Glad Bruce went with me. When we get home, he'll tell me I am right. One of the council members, Nancy, overhears me. She asks who had cancer; who am I talking about. I guess I start at that point to realize the answers to her questions are, "me" and "me." No one else. Can't wait to go home. Bruce will be there. He'll know what to do.

I don't remember too much about that night but I do remember Bruce's face. No smile, sad eyes, deep sad eyes. We just hold each other for a long time. I can't tell you if we even had supper. We talk, we cry, we plan, we cry all night long. We hold each other so close like no one or nothing can come between us or take us away or pull us apart. I guess I know now what love is all about.

I decide not to tell my family about the biopsy. After all, they aren't going to find anything. It is just a little operation and it will be over with and I will be home the same day. No big deal! Then why am I crying? Why is Bruce crying?

God is good. He put Bruce in my life. He cannot take me out of his life. Not now!

I remember seeing Bruce around City Hall off and on for several years but never really knew him until I started working for the council. So I'll start my story here.

I remember the first time I really noticed you Bruce. It was at a meeting. You were so tall and lanky. You looked like you didn't belong there or even really want to be there. Norma and Monica, my co-workers, said I should really get to know you because you were one of the good guys. But Monica wasn't sure if you were still engaged or not, so she asked. You told her you had broken off the relationship and were not seeing anyone. This was good, at least for me. We only talked for a while and then you missed a meeting and I missed seeing you. You told me you went fishing and I was jealous. You asked me if I liked fish and I said something like, "Yea, are you cooking?" I told you I liked to fish and asked you to take me with you next time. You just rolled your eyes and smiled that little smile of yours.

I remember one Friday night at Antler's Night Club. You asked me to dance and stayed by me for a little while before you told me you had to go because you were getting up early Saturday to go fishing. But I would not let you leave until you danced with me again. You picked a slow dance and you held me close. It felt so nice. I didn't want you to leave but you did.

The next Tuesday, before a council meeting, you ran into my office with a little foil package and said to put it in the refrigerator until I got home. (It was grilled tuna.) I thanked you and then you left for the meeting. I asked you again sometimes during the meeting to take me fishing.

The following Tuesday, I brought you some goose breasts and told you that you would have to cook them. I think the food exchange took place a few more times and so did our talks about fishing until one evening you asked if I wanted to go with you that Saturday. You might have been hoping I would turn you down, but I didn't. I told you we could take my boat but that you would have to check it out because it had not been used in more than a year.

You came by after work that Wednesday and I think you were pleasantly surprised that the boat was shipshape. Then we had pizza.

I was very anxious and could hardly wait until Saturday. You arrived early but I was ready. It was a beautiful October day. The fish weren't biting but we had fun. I don't talk much when I fish and I don't have to catch fish to have fun. I hoped you realized that. At one point during the day, we got out of the boat and walked on a small structure. You were so special to me. At that point, I truly wanted to kiss you.

The day ended at Black's Restaurant in Abbeville. I had no make up on and smelled like fish, but you didn't care. You brought me home and kissed me goodnight as you were leaving. I was standing in the doorway and was a little off balanced. So I made you come back and try it again. It was good!

We started seeing each other every day until you decided it was too much too fast. Maybe you just didn't trust your emotions. That only lasted about one day. Then I came down with the flu and asked you to take me to the hospital. I had a migraine and knew I would need a shot and would not be able to drive myself home. You did and you stayed with me during the whole thing and you've been with me ever since.

My kids are grown but they need me too. Their father died and I'm all that's left. They never give me any trouble, now I don't want to be a problem for them. John is married and has a child but sometimes he still needs me. Beverly is caring for her grandmother. She doesn't need another problem. I want to see my grandchild grow up.

Not now, God, not now.

March 1996

OK, the decision is made. The biopsy will be done. Am I scared? You better believe it. Dr. Carroll comes into the outpatient room and talks to us for a while before the surgery. I don't remember anything he said except that he would know something when I came out of surgery.

I kiss Bruce "good night" and say a prayer. Then the next thing I remember is Bruce's face. Without words, I know. The tears on his cheek say everything. Cancer. The big "C" word is the word that will stay with me forever.

The breast will have to be removed. The cancer is large and in an odd place and very close to the diaphragm. A large bandage is placed over the biopsy incision. I need to know more about this thing, the cancer. Who will be my oncologist? I didn't even know one. What about reconstruction? Can I just cut one breast off and have another put in all before I wake up? What kind of medicine? What type of treatment? I remember Patsy and Helen, two beautiful ladies I worked with who died of cancer. Will that be me? No, it can't be. I won't let it. Dear

God, not me. Will my whole life change? Who cares about change just as long as I have life? So many questions and not enough answers.

First, I need to tell my family. That's going to be hard. They can handle it. They've seen me go through a lot. They know I'll do whatever the doctors say.

Bruce and I know someone whose sister is an oncologist. We'll get in touch with her. That Sunday the phone rings and we are told to meet Dr. Paulette Blanchet at her office right then. On a Sunday, we meet Dr. Paulette who is also a breast cancer survivor and oncologist. She talks with us for a long time and gives us a plan of action. I need to talk to the plastic surgeon to see if he can reconstruct the breast during the removal surgery. Dr. Mes meets us after he has been in surgery all day. But my news isn't what I want to hear. Because of the location, this is not an option.

Bruce uses the Internet everyday. We talk and cry together. We hold each other. And when he holds me, I feel so lucky. God gave me something good in Bruce. He can't just end it now.

"Bruce you didn't bargain for this. There's the door. Get out while you can. No one will think badly of you. After all, we're not married. I would understand if you couldn't handle this." He looks at me with his big sad eyes, holds me tight, and says "No, not now, not ever." He stayed. This is when I really knew God gave me something special when He gave me you, Bruce. You are my strength when I am weak, my pillar to lean on, and my friend to cry with. You are my love, my life, because without you ...well, I don't want to think of that. All of this is what love is about. I try hard to only think about today, not yesterday and all its *what ifs*, not tomorrow with its *maybes* and *unknowns*. I must put all my energy into today, this very minute only. That's all any of us have.

Like the poet Ida Scott Taylor said:

One day at a time, this is enough
Do not look back and grieve on the past for it is gone
And do not be troubled about the future for it is yet to come
Live the present and make it so beautiful that it will be worth *remembering.*

Can I do this? I must. I must make memories. You do a lot of soul searching when something like this happens. I guess I never really thought about dying, just that I would be too old to care when my time to die came. But I do care. I want to live for a long time. I have so much to live for. But now Cancer is an element I had not planned on. I need to get some things together, a will, a living will, what and how I want my funeral.

No matter what anyone tells you, after the "C" word, you think of this. I want to be cremated and my ashes thrown into the sea where the sun shines on your face and the wind blows at your back. Bruce knows where this is. It's beautiful there, and it's full of memories. The music at the wake may not be conventional, but it will mean something: "Hole in the Floor of Heaven," "The Dance" by Garth Brooks, "Please Remember Me" by Tim Mc Graw, "Will You Know My Name" by Eric Clapton, "On Eagles Wings," and "The Lord's Prayer." At least that's the way I feel, something unconventional with meaning.

April 1996

Now I'm ready for my surgery and whatever else I need.

I must remember that with the tears, there must also be smiles. I must remember, like the seeds, sunshine (smiles) and rain (tears) are needed to produce a flower (life). I know I don't have to cry all the time or look sad while around my friends and people I love. They know I hurt so why remind them. I like to smile because it makes the other person smile too and the sun shines in their faces. For you Bruce, my children, family, and friends, I must remember today to smile. And I will.

The morning of my surgery comes faster than I thought. Bruce brings me to the hospital. My children, Beverly and John, come before I am brought to the operating room. Mother and Rudy just miss me and my cousin, Helen Jo, comes later. I don't remember much except there are a lot of emotions and Mother gets over excited. Helen Jo pulls her off to the side and tells her something. (Don't know what, but whatever it was worked.) Guess everyone needs a "Helen Jo" in his or her live.

I remember the tears and the faces but that's about it until Dr. Carroll comes to check the incision a day or two later. I want to look. I don't want to look. I have no idea what I will see or how I will react. Of course, I am still full of medicine and don't have my contacts in. The area is a bit swollen but it isn't that bad. I remember saying something to Dr. Carroll like he could have at least left the nipple or painted a "smiley face" on.

When I feel better, I have a talk with the hospital priest. We walk slowly and he hears my confession. He forgives me of my sins, all of them. And that is good. I feel better.

I realize now that the surgery was the easiest part. It is the mental part that afterwards is hard to deal with. Then comes the medicine with all the side effects.

Before I left the hospital I see an elderly man who has been in the room across the hall. He did not get any visitors or any flowers. And I have so many. I can't leave the hospital without saying hello and sharing my flowers. I know my friends will not mind. His eyes begin to sparkle and he smiles when I come into the room and ask if I can give him some flowers.

The flowers, cards, calls, and messages are unbelievable. I didn't know I knew that many people let alone have that many friends. But they are all there for me, some in spirit and some in person. Bruce has gone to get the car to bring me home. It takes two carts to move all my things. Someone in the hall remarks that I must be loved. They are so right. I am loved by so many, and that makes me happy and feels good. So many people go in and out of our lives but true friends last forever. And when something as big as cancer hits, you learn fast who your true friends are. They are the ones who will do whatever you let them do for you and then they want to do more. They are the ones who only see your strength when your face is green from the medicine and weak from radiation. They are the ones who cry because all they can do is look on while you suffer and know that you are the one who must endure.

Things weren't too bad for the next few weeks. After all, I had enough anti-depressants and pain pills to make anybody feel good. And I truly believed I was cancer free. The tumor and everything around it was removed. And if anything got away, chemo would kill it.

I remember one morning when I could not sleep and sitting in the living room feeling sorry for myself. After all, I had these tubes in my breast (No, not my breast, where my breast used to be.) to drain the area and keep it from getting infected. I guess reality slapped me in the face because I thought, here I am feeling sorry for myself because I have these tubes and they are going to be removed in just a few days. How shallow! There are people who have colostomy bags that cannot be removed. *Be thankful, Loretta, don't feel sorry for yourself.*

At my first visit to Dr. Carroll's office after the surgery, I have a surprise for him. Remember the smiley face? When he removed the bandage there was one under it. I thought his nurse was going to cry she was laughing so hard. And Dr. Carroll just turned red and continued his exam like nothing had happened.

Remember to Smile! I always heard if life deals you lemons, then you just make lemonade. I've got to believe and make the best of this.

May 1996

My first true outing is on a Tuesday evening, to a breast cancer support group meeting. Bruce is covering a council meeting, so he drops me off. I am going to ask somebody, anybody, I know no one at the meeting, to bring me back to City Hall. If no one can, I will just walk. It is only two blocks away. At the meeting there are about 15 ladies of all ages, early to late

20's to mid 60's. All are survivors of breast cancer. All are in different stages of their lives. I feel a little like I am at an AA meeting. But instead of saying, "Hi, my name is Jane, and I'm an alcoholic." They are saying, "Hi, my name is Judy and I've been cancer free for 3 years." And then they would say something about themselves or what happened since the last meeting.

It is my time. I proudly say, "Hi, my name is Loretta and I've been cancer free for two weeks. Two weeks! Yes, I just had surgery. Stage 2 cancer. Left breast removed. This is my first outing and, by the way, I need a ride to City Hall. Can someone bring me?" That's when I met Martha, a lovely lady with dark hair and big eyes. I remember when she introduced herself she said something about being Queen of Lymph Nodes. She had not met anyone who had as many positive nodes as she had. She drops me off at City Hall and that's when our friendship begins.

When I get to City Hall, many of the directors and co-workers are there and greet me with open arms. It feels good to be back at the office.

It was a couple of weeks later that I started my chemo, three different drugs, Methotrexate, 5 FU, and Adriamycin (the "mother" of all chemo). Two I take in the doctor's office as an IV drip and the third I wear home in a pouch for 72 hours.

Adriamycin is the one that causes hair loss. This is the one that causes me to beg for mercy. And 72 hours is a long time in hell!

Although I am given Zofran in the office before the chemo to help with the nausea, it is gone by the next day. I planned my chemo for Fridays so that, if I had problems, I wouldn't miss too much work. But what I didn't realize was that if I had problems, the doctor's office would be closed on weekends too. I didn't know to go the hospital and that they could give me something that would help. So as the day progressed, the sicker I got. I am nauseated but can't throw up. I just dry heave. The bathroom floor is my buddy. It is cool and I just lie there, just in case. Nothing helps. Oh God! Just let me throw up and I'll feel better. I can feel my energy leaving. I don't have the energy nor the will to move and I don't care.

I know I have to eat and drink but just the thought of food is repulsive. I need to throw up but nothing comes up. And, the smell, the smell of food makes it worse. Bruce tries everything. Anything I think I want, he gets for me. Then when I get it, I can't get it down. My head hurts from heaving so much. Is this normal? Will this be every time? "Bruce, please don't cook anything." The smell, Oh God, I can't handle the smell of food. And yet I know I must eat. But the taste, it just tastes like metal. I can truly taste the fork. (I never thought to use a plastic fork. That might have helped.)

That whole weekend I could feel myself getting weaker. By Monday morning, Bruce has me packed and in the car to get to Dr. Paulette's office early. I am given something that settles everything down and makes me sleepy. Joan, Dr. Paulette's nurse, finishes up my chemo and unplugs me from my mediport (the thing that looks like a growth under my skin where I receive my chemo). I go home and sleep for what seems like days. Then, back to work. I work as much as I can. Some days are only for an hour or two. But that's okay. I do what I can and my co-workers (Thank you) pick up the rest. But working takes my mind off of what's happening. The only thing is, my mind isn't always working right. My co-workers have to proofread everything I do. Guess the chemo messes with the good cells as well as the bad.

On the tenth day after my chemo, my hair starts to fall out. I have already bought a wig (you must call it a cranial prosthesis for insurance purposes) that looks just like my hair. So I am not too upset. After all, my hair is already very short. The transition shouldn't be hard, right? Wrong!

It doesn't take long once the hair starts falling. A little here and a little there, in the bed and on my pillow, all over my clothes, at work, on the table, and everywhere. It sticks to me when I take a bath. I can go outside and run my hands over my head and hand full of hair falls. I never knew I had that much hair. I can't handle it any longer. It is terrible. I get the scissors and ask Bruce to just cut off what is left. He looks at me with a look of fear and says, "But what if I mess it up?" *My God, mess what up?* How can he mess this up? It is already a mess. I am serious. It is going one way or another. And if I have to, I will do it myself. I run to the bathroom (that seemed to be my haven these days) and am about to cut off what little is left of my hair myself. At that point, Bruce comes in and takes the scissors away from me and asks if I am sure. He cuts my hair. After all the hair is gone, I am better. I still cry because now you really can tell I have cancer. No matter what I do, I am bald and no matter what, I have cancer. (You know, you may lose the hair on your head, eyebrows and eyelashes, the hair under your arms and legs, and the hair all over your body. You may lose all this hair, but the hair over your upper lip <u>never</u> falls out.)

Yes, now the cancer is really there. Even with the loss of one breast, the hair loss is more disturbing. I can stuff a bra and put a shirt on and no one will know. But the hair...I'll wear a wig or put on a scarf or hat and still everyone knows something is wrong. Then when you lose your eyebrows and lashes, no amount of make-up can really help. But you try. My skin color is different, almost greenish white. I buy new make-up to try to add color back to my face. (Sometimes you lose all your body hair and sometimes you don't.) From the waist down, I look more like a young girl before puberty. From the waist up, and depending on which side you are looking at, I look like a little old man on the left (no breast/no hair) and on the right, a little old lady (saggy breast/no hair). *My God, has my body turned on me?* It was always there for me. My breasts were fairly large, my waist was small, and my legs were firm. Now my ribs show. I have only one breast and because of the kind of cancer I have, that one will be going soon. I feel so weak. *My God, My God, have you forsaken me?*

Today is the day I put on my wig. What will people say? "My you look good"..."I like your HAIR"...Does this mean that I had been looking bad and my real hair was really a mess? They are only trying to be nice. But I hate this wig. I hate what it stands for. I hate everything about it. It gets in my way - just like cancer. It changes my whole appearance - just like cancer. It replaces the good - just like cancer. I hate it. I hate it - just like cancer.

Get a grip, Loretta. If you hate it that much, then do something about it - just like you are doing with cancer. So I do! I give it my best shot!! I give the wig away and start wearing scarves and hats. (Now I really do mean hats - big ones, small ones, straw ones, felt ones, fishing hats, cowboy hats, ball caps. You name it; I wore it.) I decide I am going to make the best of it. Everyone who knows me knows my hair is gone. They don't care. So let's dress it up. Everyday I can be someone different. (Maybe a movie star, a cowgirl, no one knew what I would wear next.) Those who don't know about the cancer may just think I am making a fashion statement! *You've just got to do what you got to do, whatever gets you through the day. You've just got to do it!*

June 1996

It is during the "hat" days that I meet Neppie. Like Martha, it is at a support group meeting. She and her daughter (you could hardly tell who was the mother and who was the daughter) are at the meeting. She sits very still and does not say much. (I do remember how sad Neppie's eyes looked.) I ask for her phone number and give her mine. (We've been talking every since.)

Everyone going through cancer needs someone who's been there too. You need someone to tell you that it's just the medicine that makes you feel this way or it's going to do that or you might feel like this, or it's okay to cry, it's okay to be scared, it's okay to throw up because food smells. All of this will pass but you need to keep your strength up, so eat a baked potato. They don't smell if you microwave them. And they don't have much taste when you eat them. But they can be your life support

for food. And when you feel sorry for yourself, that's okay too.
No one told me this. I just had to find out myself.

My protocol is six treatments. Each one makes me a little
weaker than the one before. Just as I start to feel better, it's time
for another. My guts burn from the chemo. My skin is sensitive
to the sun. There are times I go into the doctor's office to get
something to help and I know I must look green. I sure feel like
it. I lie across the chair. I don't care. *Just give me something,*
anything. Please just make the nausea and this burn in my
stomach go away. It seems like my life is just fading away
treatment by treatment. But it is going to get better. It has to. I
have too many things to do, people to meet, places to go...I have
my family and friends and Bruce. God has been good to me up
to this point. Now what is He doing, what is He thinking? He
must have made a mistake mixing me up with someone else! I
know that there is a certain amount of hurt that must be felt in
this world. Maybe I'm stronger than others, maybe my faith will
get me through this. *One day at a time Loretta, remember that's*
all any of us have. Life does exist after cancer.

July 1996

The sun is too hot for me to get out while I'm taking my
treatments. It just drains me of any energy I have. So this

summer I will do exactly what the doctors says. Fishing, biking, hiking, and boating are all on the back burner. I vow I will do all these things as soon as I can.

Mother cooks the whole summer and each time she comes to visit she brings me food. All my friends do the same. I guess they think I am going to starve. (After all I have dropped from a size 10 to a size 2.) Or maybe they think food is fuel for the soul.

August 1996

It seems like a lifetime but by the end of August I have taken my last treatment. All my test results are good. The Cancer is gone. Almost as soon as I stop the chemo, my energy gets better and my hair starts growing back. (Although, when I look at all our vacation and fishing pictures, I do not have hair. Just a scarf and hat.)

One evening at the support group, we start talking about reconstruction, pros/cons, do's/don'ts. It was about 50/50. Martha says she is satisfied with her surgery and if she has to do it again, she'd make them bigger. Then there is a lady who says she had her implants removed because she couldn't feel her children hug her. Martha's doctor is the same one I am seeing. After the meeting, she calls me over and we talk a little while.

Then she says, "Here, you want to see?" Up comes the shirt and there they are. I don't know what I was expecting. But I'm sure this was not it. They aren't anatomically correct but with clothes on, they look fine.

As soon as my blood counts are up, I prepare for my reconstruction. Dr. Mes talks to Bruce and me about removing the other breast and the affect it could have even on a relationship. But our relationship is strong. And I am determined the Cancer isn't going to attack the other breast.

The surgery is a success. No breasts, no cancer, just implants. They look like Martha's, not anatomically correct but I guess I'll get used to them. Every week for about a month, I go in for saline adjustments until the right size is reached. Then we wait for the skin to stretch and I have the final work done and a nipple tattooed on my left breast. The doctor left the nipple on the right one. I decide on a tattoo instead of a nipple made from the skin of the groin area. I don't want to be cut on again.

I guess it was about the time I took off my hat that the celebration really began and Bruce asked me to marry him. I remember thinking he said he would never leave me and I guess he really meant it. "But Bruce, are you sure? After all, I buried two husbands. My track record is not that great. And now, there's Cancer and artificial breasts. Are you sure?"

October 1996

It is just a simple ceremony in the back yard with friends. Even the judge is one of our friends. They are the only ones who know what our plans are. After the wedding we invited friends and co-workers to what most of them think is a surprise party for Bruce. His birthday is this week. Some suspect but all are surprised when I show up in white (never wore white before) and the license is the first thing they see when they walk in. It is great. Boy, am I happy, and proud; proud that Bruce chose me as his wife; but prouder still of my hair. Now, picture this, Bruce is losing the hair on top of his head and I'm growing some. When we sign our marriage license, one of our friends takes our picture. And you know what, we look just alike, hair-wise! My head shines just as much as his.

After the party, we take off for North Carolina stopping at Bruce's folks. Bruce keeps flashing his ring. He becomes left-handed. But his folks never say a thing. He can't stand it any more, so he just busts out with the news. His dad jumps up from his chair and gives me a big hug and his mother just smiles the biggest smile ever. I do believe they like me! I remember calling my family from an old inn in North Carolina. Beverly and John are a little disappointed that they weren't at the ceremony. But being the great kids that they are, they are very excited for me. Mom and Rudy are concerned but pleased also. They all know I am happy. A couple sitting nearby must have heard me because, when I hung the phone up, they congratulate me and wish us the best.

Fall 1996

For the next few months, life is beautiful. We fish, hike, bike, and all the things we did before "C." I am feeling good about myself and everything is going fine.

I make the decision to have the final part of my reconstructive work done the first of March (one year after the cancer diagnosis.)

January 1997

One January weekend we decide to go fishing. The weather will be great and the fish are biting. We start loading the boat which Bruce parks conveniently under the carport so I don't have to walk far. I never was very graceful and don't do two things at once very well. And I hit my head on a cross beam so hard it knocks me down and knocks my cap off. We go fishing but the pain in my neck doesn't get better. It is so bad by Sunday that I sleep in while Bruce catches fish!

I hurt but don't know what doctor to see. I know something is wrong. The pain in my neck is like no other I have had. It is different than when I injured it in a car wreck years ago. My doctors say all my cancer tests are normal, not to worry, it is just a whiplash and with time and therapy I will be all right. I swim, and it hurts. I go to therapy, and it hurts. I have therapeutic massages, and it hurts. Something's wrong, I know it. The doctors are willing to bet their salaries that it is just whiplash. But it still hurts. I am due to undergo reconstruction and need chest x-rays. So the doctors decide, just to satisfy me, they will order a neck x-ray.

March 1997

All things come to a halt. Something's wrong. The operation is on hold because the doctors see something. Part of the bone, third cervical vertebrae, is gone. I am sent to another doctor. I am already upset and he just looks at the x-ray and says, "Yea, it is cancer. My sister had this and she died." Gee Thanks Doc! That's just what I want to hear. Bruce and I leave his office so upset that we forget to pick up the x-rays. And they have never been seen since. They are lost in the paperwork at someone's office. Guess I should have taken the doctors up when they were willing to bet their salaries it wasn't cancer!

More tests, more doctors. This time I'm picking the doctor. I see Dr. Bertuccini, my neurosurgeon and I see my plastic surgeon again. I go to Shreveport to see a specialist, Dr. Weinberger, who talks to us about a risky stem cell transplant procedure, sometimes called a bone marrow transplant. At this point in my life, I feel I have no choice but to undergo this risky procedure. My treatment is now planned.

I first need a biopsy of the area of my neck. Because of the location of the cancer near the spinal cord, a needle biopsy cannot be done. It is going to be a surgical biopsy.

Cancer, yes. Metastatic Breast Cancer. *How can that be? I don't have any breasts.* This isn't good. This is the first time I hear the word death and that it could happen if we don't take drastic measures. Do it. Do whatever it takes. Just don't let me die. I don't want to die, I can't die, I will not. It's not fair. Not again. Hold Me, Bruce. Hold Me.

I just read something I wrote what seems to be a long time ago, but it was just last year. I wrote how scared I was when I first was told I had cancer. How panic-stricken and frightened I was when I realized this was now my life. That devastating feeling seemed to have diminished over time. But now, it is back, trying to re-surface. I must not let that feeling over take my life. I must remember what I wrote when I was first diagnosed with cancer:

> *"I'm not a quitter*
> *I am a fighter*
> *I will survive!!"*

But I would be lying to you if I said I'm not scared.

Mother always told me I was hardheaded and I guess I have always run head on into brick walls all my life only to bounce back, get up, dust myself off, and try again. Things would go fine for a while, and then the cycle would start over again, hit that wall, bounce back, get up, dust myself off, and try again. Using this analogy, you might say my first brick wall was my relationship with my mother. Growing up wasn't easy. Guess it never is when you are an only child and your mother is a single parent. I never knew my father and he never saw me. He was a soldier in the Army, died serving our country, and received the Purple Heart and a Silver Star posthumously. I now know she did the best she could with what she had to work with, me, a hardheaded, headstrong daughter. We butted heads more than once, but I would bounce back and go on with my life. Married and two children later, I buried my first husband. That wall was hard. It was the first time that I truly felt alone and had to do for my children and myself. *Bounce back, Loretta, pick yourself up, and start over again.*

Things were going pretty good for a long time. I remarried, saw my first grandchild born, then I buried my second husband. There was that wall again, but this time I knew I could do it on my own and bounce back.

Things were looking up, new job, and a great man in my life. Brick wall ...Cancer. This wasn't supposed to happen to me. *As before, Loretta, pick yourself up, dust yourself off, and go forward.*

Life looks good, married again. Cancer again. Brick wall again. Again I'll pick myself up, dust myself off, and go on and go as many times as I have to. If I hit that wall again, maybe it will crumble and fall or maybe it will ultimately do me in. But whichever the case may be, and until that time, I'll keep bouncing back, get up, dust myself off, and go on with my life. Again.

"Cancer may have robbed me of that blissful ignorance that once led me to believe that tomorrow stretched forever. In exchange, I've been granted the wisdom to see each today as something special, a gift to be used wisely and fully. Nothing can take that away. Hopes and dreams reign where cancer cannot go." This was an email titled, "A Cancer Survivor," the author, I do not know.

I remember leaving the doctor's office after being told my cancer was back. I remember feeling sorry for myself until I saw a man with no legs and I thanked God that that was not me. All you have to do is look around and find someone worse off than you.

Okay doctors; let's get this battle started. I want this war over. Load your guns, doc. I'm ready for round two!

I know if we don't kill the cancer, it will just keep surfacing. I don't want to live my life waiting for the next time. I am basically healthy and the cancer is in a place that we can deal with, this time.

Bruce, you are my strength when I am weak, my calm when I am frantic. You literally bring music into my life. The kinds of music that mellow you out and make you appreciate the soft, precious things in life. You taught me how to reach deep inside and pull out what I need to get through the day. Now keep reminding me to dig deeper because I know I'm going to need more.

Dr. Bertuccini puts me in a neck brace because I am now missing part of the bone at the third cervical vertebrae. I hate wearing it. It reminds me of my feelings with the wig. This is my cancer. This is what I feel. After all, the cancer itself never hurt. It just hides its face and destroys. I don't want to wear this neck brace. I look sick. Oh my God, listen to me. My life is on the line here and all I can think of is what I look like. Am I that shallow of a person? Is that my problem? *Get over it Loretta, dig deeper. Think of why he ordered that brace. Think of that man with no legs. Think Loretta. You can get, and will get, over this. It's for your own good.*

The doctors tell me that this cancer probably will recur in other bones unless preventive treatment is used. They say having cancer in the bone is not as severe as the more difficult to treat cancer of the liver or lungs, but aggressive therapy is required because my cancer metastasized in less than a year's time. The doctors say this protocol is the most aggressive form. If all goes as anticipated, they are hopeful that radiation will result in a stronger vertebrae and that surgery may not be required to fuse the affected bone in my neck. We have to rid the neck of the cancer before it destroys more bone. Dr. Noel's staff gives me a few blue freckles to mark the spots for the radiation and then one round every day for six weeks. This doesn't hurt and I only have a bit of a sore throat. I can handle this.

May 1997

The chemo that comes next is different, Ifosfamide and Cisplatin, a form of platinum. Because of its intensity, I must go to the hospital for infusions of two rounds, four days each session with approximately three to four weeks rest between the two doses. This has to be done before I go to Shreveport for my high dosage of chemotherapy and stem cell replacement treatments. This stuff really hurts and makes me sick. Sicker than the other chemo and what little hair I have coming in, I lose again. Every part of my body feels like it is on fire and I can't put it out. I hurt so bad. "God, make it go away. I'll be good. I'll do whatever you want just make it stop hurting. It burns inside."

I don't want anyone to see me like this, especially my mother and kids. I don't know what I would do if I had to watch my children suffer like this. I'm sorry Mother. I don't mean to make you worry about me.

Between the two treatments I get to go home. Just being home helps. I don't like the hospital. It smells of death. Just as soon as I start feeling better, I have to go back to the hospital again. I have to do it all over again. I worry over every little ache and pain asking myself if that might be cancer too.

I've got to go through one more round of chemo. *Dig, Loretta, reach deep. You have to stay healthy.* It burns. My guts are on fire and now I'm constipated. Are my organs shutting down? Am I going to die? *Get a hold of yourself Loretta. Just take an enema. It's just the chemo and all the pain pills. You haven't eaten that much. You're not going to die.*

Well, you're going to be okay. The Cisplatin leaves me weak and hurting. I return to my old friend, the bathroom floor.

My white counts are too low to go to Shreveport and they need to be up. I have to take some medicine called Neupogen to stimulate my bone marrow, twice before Shreveport. It makes my bones hurt. But it works.

I had heard about a priest in a small town south of here who heals people. I went to his healing service with a friend, Allyson. All I did was cry. I went back the next week to talk with him before I go to Shreveport. Ted, my neighbor and a cancer patient, and I go together. I told Ted, "Just looking at us, we are the healthiest looking two sick people in Lafayette." I want the priest to hear my confession, forgive me of my sins, and heal me of my cancer. He hears my confession but doesn't forgive me of my sins. Bruce and I weren't married in the Church. Therefore, he can't give me absolution. He says maybe my parish priest could but he could not. He wants Bruce to have his previous marriages annulled. Then we can get married in the Church. Now I have a problem with this. If the Catholic Church does not think you are married unless you are married in the Catholic Church, then why do you need to have something annulled that does not exist in the first place? And anyway, I don't believe in annulments. Why should I cause the families of his ex-wives to be troubled for something I don't believe in? But most important, in my heart I know God put Bruce in my life at this time for a reason. A reason far greater than any man will ever know. I pray to God everyday, we talk everyday, He forgives me everyday, and everyday I thank Him for all His blessings. If God forgives me, so too should this man.

June 1997

I guess we leave Lafayette thinking Shreveport is going to be the answer to our prayers. We bring my dog Pepper to Bruce's parents. They have been great through all this and have done whatever they can to help. I've never been away from Pepper for more than a week. This is going to be over a month. He'll probably think I have deserted him. Monica and her husband, Marcus, will check on the house. Marcus added more security to the house alarm system. Allyson will look after my little garden and John will mow the lawn. Mother bought me t-shirts and sweats for the hospital. Bruce packed his fishing rod so he could go fishing on the days he could break away. Guess I'm ready.

It's a typical June in Louisiana, hot and humid. Guess I should be glad I don't have to be outside. But I wish I were outside. I meet a man while waiting to see the doctor. His eyes are red and swollen. He tells me his wife isn't doing well. The doctors just told them her cancer had spread to the brain. She had breast cancer and had been fighting recurrence in the liver, lungs, and bones for over three and a half years. How do you console someone who must feel all that he loves and holds dear is dying a little at a time and there is nothing he can do to make it better? I must remember that we are all in God's hands. I must remember that and know in my heart that I must go through this and maybe for this lady and her husband, maybe for others, maybe just for myself. My prayers are to be strong, that I don't disappoint God, and that I am cured and free of cancer.

Here in the hospital, things start to move fast. My veins aren't very prominent and they have problems administering an I.V. which is to be used for the medicine I will need to help minimize the side effects. There are about three interns and one doctor trying to get a main line into a vein in my neck. The skin is first numbed and then an intern tries to find the vein in my neck. It hurts; she misses and is still tying to get the needle into the vein. She can't. I can't stand the pain any longer. "Please stop!" The doctor takes over and after several tries, the main line is in. It looks like something is growing out of my neck. This is where the doctors and nurses will remove my stem cells, give me chemo, and then return the cells back to me. This is also where they will feed me when I get too weak and sick to eat and drink.

The procedure is referred to as an autologous bone marrow transplant. It is actually the removal of ones own stem cells, the basis of red and white blood cells and platelets. They are more mature than cells in the bone marrow. The chemo that I will be receiving will be so strong that it will wipe out my immune system. Using my own cells will restore my immune system and is not as risky as using a donor's cells. Remember this is a transplant procedure. Your body could reject a donor's cells just like it could reject a donor heart. Because the cells are mine and clinically free of cancer at this point, I have a better chance that my body will not reject the cells. The machine used to harvest the cells looks and sounds like a washing machine. The nurses will draw my blood through the main line. It will travel through this machine, separate, and the whole blood will be returned to me. The stem cells will be checked, tested, counted, and then frozen until it's time to return them to me. Again, using the main line.

I can tell this is not easy on Bruce, especially when they miss a vein and every time it hurts. I am given Benadryl to help with side effects, but it makes me frantic and I wiggle like a worm. I cannot stay still. It doesn't calm me down. It just makes me wiggle. But it doesn't take long for them to draw the amount of stem cells I will need to do the two procedures, two hours and it's over.

The next day, they start my treatment. This is my first high-dose chemotherapy consisting of Taxol and Melphalan. Because these drugs wipe out the immune system, I will have to spend the next four weeks in a special facility sanitized with purified air and may have to wear a surgical mask to prevent contacting germs. Infusion of blood and platelets will be needed. The chemo makes me sick. My energy is gone. I have to wash my mouth out with three different washes to help keep the "crud" down. The mouth sores come anyway because my immune system is so weak and it makes it impossible to eat, drink, and talk. This is the only thing in my life that has stopped me from eating and talking. So you know it's bad. They feed me through the tubes in my neck. I don't care. I'm too weak to care anymore.

All I want to do is sleep. My eyes don't focus. And I brought my computer to do work. What a joke!

I am given two rounds of steroids to help with some of the side effects of the Taxol. I can't concentrate, just sleep. They weigh me every day to make sure my body's not retaining too much fluid. It's hard to stand up and get on the scales. The nurses have to help sometimes. And sometimes I am given Lasix to get rid of the fluid.

While I sleep, Bruce goes to check out a lake. That's good. It'll get his mind off this. He also found a place to go exercise.

Wish I could go too. They have a bike up here and soon I'm supposed to walk the halls, or ride the bike, up to a mile a day to get my strength back. *They must be crazy, I can't even hold my head up and they want me to walk.*

I'm so sick now. The chemo has my blood counts zeroed out. I feel very close to death. I never really wondered what it would be like to die, until now. You just lay there, you don't move, you can't move, you don't want to move. You can't eat; you don't care about anything. All your energy is gone. Bruce took some pictures of me and of the hospital room and stuff. He won't let me see them. Maybe it's because I do look like I'm dying. This feeling was affirmed at one of my visits back in Shreveport after my first round of transplants. Dr. Weinberger said he brought me as close to death as he could get me only to bring me back again. This was his way of killing the cancer.

It was during this lowest point in my treatment, I guess you might say the most critical, that something very special took place. One night a hand on my left shoulder awakens me. I thought it was Bruce because he was sleeping on his mat on that side of the bed. But he was still asleep. It wasn't a nurse. The door to my room and all the equipment the nurses monitored was to my right. But I know I felt a hand and no one else was in the room. I went back to sleep only to be awakened again by a hand on my left shoulder. I was aware that no one could have been there because the way the hand held my shoulder the person would have had to be behind my bed and up against the wall. This did not scare me, I just went back to sleep. It was like I recognized the hand. It was a strong hand, but gentle, like my first husband's hand. It was the last thing I saw of him when I identified his body after his accident. For the next several days I became more aware of what was happening. The hand, again on my left shoulder, woke me up. I felt it was there to tell me I was being watched over. And that's when I realized I was not alone. My angels were with me. I saw them all at the foot of my bed watching over me and smiling. Larry, Kevin, Daddy, Uncle Bevo, Uncle George, Paw Paw, Helen, Patsy, Grandma and Grandpa, and some others that I did not know. They were there for what felt about three or four days. Then one day, when I was getting better and my blood counts started going up, they each touched me. I felt angel wings brush against my face and then they were gone. I guess you might say angels, my guardian angels, kissed me. I felt at peace.

I remember a dream I had not too long ago, before the big "C." In it I saw Larry, my first husband and he told me to be careful that the road ahead would be rough. Then after the diagnosis of cancer, I had another dream in which Larry visited me again. Before he left he told me he would see me soon. I didn't understand then but I do now. I have seen him in a dream once since his visit in the hospital. I had been diagnosed with cancer for the third time, about a year and a half after that hospital visit. He told me he did not have time to visit; he had other things to do. Did this mean I was going to be all right and that he must be with someone who needed him more? I hope so! God appears to us in many ways. We just need to pay attention. And through my angels, I saw Him.

July 1997

My stay in the hospital lasted one month. Then I went home. Home. You don't know how good that is. I don't do much for the next three weeks but sleep. My energy level is zero and all my counts are low but climbing. I am thinking about trying to go back to work, if only for a few hours a day. I am not sure if I am ready. But there was that day when the phone went out. You must understand, living in the country, you don't get visitors who are just in the neighborhood so they thought they would drop by to see you. They make an appointment. I don't get many visitors during the week so the phone line is my lifeline to civilization. And when it went out, I was lost. It was only out 24 hours and some of that time I was asleep. But when the phone man came by, I truly wanted to kiss him. That's when I knew it was time for me to go back to work.

September 1997

By the time I was strong enough to work eight hours a day, it was time to go back to Shreveport for my second transplant and round of chemo. This time it would be Cytoxan, Thiotepa, and Carboplatin. I am ready. I have my PETScan and it is clean. A PETScan is a fairly new piece of equipment and more responsive than a MRI or Bone Scan. At this time, Shreveport is the only place in Louisiana that has one. And it shows no signs of cancer. So if there are any little cells left, I feel confident that this last treatment will zap them.

I swear I must glow in the dark. I am given a radioactive drug for my bones that actually set off a Geiger counter. The other medicine is just as bad as the first but I am determined that I will get through this and everything will be fine.

Bruce and I celebrate our first anniversary in the hospital between chemo and stem cells. Not exactly my choice of places to go and things to do on your first anniversary! But we did it, one year and many more to come.

I knew the second round of chemo could be more difficult than the first because I was still so weak. It had only been three months since the first stem cell procedure and my body had not fully recovered. But I guess I wasn't really prepared for what took place next.

Then one night, I remember Bruce waking me and telling me to eat a popsicle. A nurse is wiping me down with alcohol. I don't want that damn popsicle. I just want to sleep. Why did he wake me up? The nurses wake me up every two hours to check my vitals and now Bruce is waking me up to eat a popsicle. What are you doing? Then I see that look in his eye and know something is wrong but all I want to do is sleep and they won't let me. When I ask what is wrong, Bruce says my fever is up and they have to get it down and eating that damn popsicle would help. While the nurse bathes me with alcohol and places ice around my body, she continues to monitor my fever. I later learned it was 106^0. I started eating popsicles but I also was losing control of my body functions. That was the first time I felt I had no control over what was happening. Bruce keeps feeding me and helps the nurse clean me up just to wash me down again. I don't know how long this went on but it must have been the biggest part of the night. But when the fever dropped, they let me sleep and continued monitoring me.

Now the doctor tells me to call in all my sources. I am going to need whole blood and platelets. And I know prayers, too. I call Neppie and a prayer line is started. Bruce calls John and between he and Beverly they gather a dozen or so people who drive to Shreveport the next day. Bruce, John, and someone else are my platelet donors. (I met this lady one day about a year later while visiting John in De Ridder. I couldn't thank her enough. She was just glad to see me up and going which was a lot different than when she saw me before.) The screening of blood is very intense. I don't remember too much of the next few days. My fever is still there around 100-102^0. That's not too bad. I am on antibiotics and am told the infection is from bacteria we all have in our body. Mine just went berserk and started attacking my body that is unable to fight back because of my weak immune system. It wasn't until later, after I went home, that I saw a documentary on stem cell replacement. In the documentary, they mentioned this type of bacteria and said sometimes it kills. If I had known that, what would I have done? I don't know. All I know is even after I come home the fever goes back up to 102^0. I am told to go immediately to the hospital where they start me on an intravenous antibiotic administered every four hours. My veins are bad and they are having problems. The line used in Shreveport to administer medicine had been removed and now they are considering another. The anesthesiologist tries but I am so dehydrated that he is unable to find a site. So it is back to my arm and keeping my fingers crossed that a vein will last for at least four hours. Back home the nurses are coming round the clock every four hours. This is going to last until my fever is gone. I take my temperature every 2-4 hours and hope that the next time it won't be over 100^0.

Finally, after two weeks, it is 99^0 and holding. Then it's down to normal and I start feeling better.

November 1997

After about another three weeks, I start back to work and by Thanksgiving I am full time. Thanksgiving, boy do I know the true meaning of that word. And yes, I have a lot to be thankful for, a good husband, beautiful children, lovely grandchildren (a new little granddaughter was born Thanksgiving week.), great parents and in-laws, and a tremendous extended family and friends. These are the things important in live, not money or material things. It's the ones you love and love you in return. Life is great. God is good.

When we left Shreveport this last time, the doctor told us that this did not mean I would never have cancer again and, that in all probability, I could have a recurrence in about ten years. I decided ten years was a long time and that by then a cure might be a reality. So I was going to live as normal a life as I could. After all, there were several ladies I met along the way that did not make it through this treatment. I was just one of the lucky ones.

December 1998 – March 1999

For the next year and a half, my husband took me to new places and we did things I had not done before. I caught the biggest redfish I've ever caught, 40 pounds, night fishing near the jetties. With no hair, wearing a cap, and no makeup on, Bruce took pictures of me fighting the fish and then landing it. We let him go after the trophy picture was taken. And then there was the surprise when Bruce did an article and there I was in the middle of "Louisiana Sportsman" magazine.

We biked, we hiked, and we lived life to the fullest. After my last treatment, we bought a camper to see the countryside. I played with the grandchildren. I flew to Florida with Beverly and Evie to visit my Mother and Rudy. We vacationed in North Carolina, in Big Bend, Texas, and crossed the border into Mexico. All and all life was great. I even adopted Rudy as my Dad, legal papers and all.

Now, I have very few problems. But I'll be honest with you; every problem, every bruise, every pain, and every something different, I just know it is cancer. But my scans are fine. My blood work is good. But then there was one blood test that just started to elevate a little each time. I really got concerned when I came across the results of the same test done the year before and the numbers had doubled. I go into a panic mode. I want some answers and I don't feel like I am getting them. So I ask for a PETScan again. I am frightened but determined I am going to find out what's happening.

My gut instinct says cancer and my heart says no. But I know before the doctor says anything. I know something is wrong. When Dr. Lillian comes to get Bruce and me, I see it in his face. I remember him saying he wasn't good at this but had to tell me the cancer was back or maybe it never really left. There is a place in my neck and another on my right rib. This isn't what I want to hear but I know it is there. *Sometimes your gut knows.* Bruce and I leave the office and as soon as we walk outside, we cry. We hold each other and just cry. This has got to be the last time!

Okay folks! This is it. I don't plan to get sick again. So I'm taking a different approach. Besides traditional medicine, I am going to see Dr. Jester, a doctor of Eastern medicine. He had cancer 12 years ago and was told he had only three months to live. He had heard of a hospital in the East that cured people with traditional Eastern medicine. He was cured and started studying and practicing Eastern medicine in Lafayette. So here I am, the East meets the West. Maybe now, this cancer has met its match.

April 1999 – February 2000

Now I'm taking all new (Western) IV drugs, Herceptin, Aridia, and Arimidex. Herceptin is giving once a week and Aridia, once a month. Arimidex is a pill taken once a day. It's a good thing I have insurance. Herceptin is about $1,600 a week and Aridia is about $1,000 a month. I figured, at this rate, I have 25 years before my insurance plays out. That's if I stay healthy. At this point, I will receive these drugs for the rest of my life or until something better comes along. And who knows, it may.

Then there are the Eastern herbs. I take a powder three times a day and 11 pills three times a day. I rattle when I walk, but at least I get my daily intake of fluid taking these pills. One of the herbs is to help keep my counts up while taking chemo. The others are to build my immune system, redirect my DNA and T-cells to kill the cancer.

Dr. Bertuccini has me back in the neck brace while I'm in a vehicle. He has me so scared. He told me that if something happens and the bone in my neck breaks, I would be left paralyzed. He once told me that football players perform with less bone than this, but how? And I seem to hit my head all the time. I've hit it on the camper door, the car door, Bruce's elbow, you name it, and I've hit it there. Guess it's good to have a hard head. Although, Dr. Bert reminds me, it's not the head he's concerned about, it's the neck.

Today is Monday. I don't really look forward to Mondays anymore because every Monday I take my medicine. Every Monday I get stuck. Every Monday strange medicine is put into my veins doing God-knows-what to my body. But they say it kills the cancer. I pray it kills the cancer and doesn't just make it hide. *Please God kill this cancer. I'm tired of all this. It's time for the cancer to die.*

Some days I just don't want to do this any more. That doesn't mean I'm giving up. It just means I don't want to have to do this any more! The medicine makes my bones hurt. I feel like I have the flu all the time. It doesn't get better and my energy is getting low again. No one really knows how much I hurt at work. I just know I have got to keep up the front. Sometimes it's hard to put on a happy face, but no one needs to know. Dr. Jester put me on an herb to help with the energy. I cry a lot when I get real tried and because it hurts so much. Dr. Paulette prescribes Paxil and Celebrex for depression and pain. They seem to help although Celebrex makes my stomach feel strange.

My muscles are tight and I have little stamina. I've tried exercising again but I hurt too much. Dr. Paulette now has me at physical therapy doing exercise in the water. I sure hope this works.

I don't want to go to the doctor. Every doctor I go to gives me bad news. Now things are looking up. My tumor markers are within the normal range. *Normal. Now that's a word I haven't heard in a long time.* Looking back, my markers haven't been this low in years. *Does that mean the medicines are working? I guess it does.* All I know is that the day I called the doctor's office and Joan told me my markers were 30, you could hear me down the hall at work and I'm still excited. This is a blessing. God has blessed me once more.

I don't know if it's just mental or truly physical, but I feel better than ever. Of course my neck still bothers me, but I feel better. I don't ask myself if it's the medicine, if it's the herbs, or if it's the prayers, or just all three. I just know God has given me a little longer on this earth for some reason I do not know. I only know I pray a lot more than I used to. I carry my rosary in the car and instead of listening to the radio, I say those beads. I also have found a friend in Charlene Richard, the Cajun saint. I visit her grave and ask her to pray to Jesus for me. Whatever is happening to me is good, both mentally as well as physically. And life is beautiful and God is good. And it's all right.

I had a sinus cold the other day. And you know what? I knew it was just a sinus cold. Not, "Oh my God has the cancer spread to my sinuses?" I truly knew it was just a sinus cold. I think if this had happened last year, I would be at the doctor's asking for tests to be done and what was going on. But, although it may not always be easy to do, I'm not running to the doctor because I've had sinus problems before, I'll have them again, and I know I'll get over it just like I've done before. Okay, I still hurt. I still have pains, but I'll get over them.

March 2000

My how time flies when you're having fun! Now it's March again. If I can only make it through March this year I'll be okay.

But now I'm looking at my tumor markers, again. And again, they are going up. I insist on another PETScan. And as I feared, the cancer is still there. It was just hiding and now it has spread to some lymph nodes in my chest, on some ribs, and back in my neck. Arimidex is stopped and Taxotere is added to my weekly routine. With all the new medicines, all the new studies, all the money, science, and effort, why hasn't someone found a cure for this cancer? (Why don't doctors tell their patients more about trial studies and alternative medicines?)

Dr. Paulette has been trying to get me to retire, but I'm not ready. She even wrote a letter to the retirement system on my behalf. The day I received a copy of this letter, I came unglued.

Now I know that metastasis breast cancer is not curable, at least not yet. I know that the cancer in my neck is in a critical location. I know all this. But to see it in writing is another thing. The letter stated: that I suffered from <u>terminal cancer</u> and that the sites of my disease would eventually <u>paralyze</u> me and cause my <u>death</u>. I cried for days until I realized that <u>everyone is terminal</u>. No one gets out of here alive. Everyone will die.

May 2000

So, I'm still going to work, but it's so hard now. I have very little energy. It takes everything I have just to get up and get dressed in the morning. I will not complain. I will not give up. I am not a quitter. I am a fighter. I <u>know</u> I will survive. But this is tough, four years tough. When will it end? I feel so tired. *Okay, Loretta, get dressed and go to work. You can do it. You can do it. You can...*

I can't. I'm too tired to do anything else. I go to work later now than before and sometimes leave early. Now all my doctors think I should stop working. But I am not a quitter. Let me just lie on the couch for a little while. Bruce thought I would feel more comfortable if I took my shoes off. I'm too tired to even do that. "If you want them off, you take them off." Then there was: not tonight Bruce, sorry kids I'm too tired, maybe next weekend, I have to work. This isn't fair, not for me, not for my family, not even for my job.

I'll try again to go to work today. Today will be different. But it isn't. I'm so tired. I walk into my boss's office and say, "Lloyd, I can hardly put one foot in front of the other. I just can't do this anymore."

Those were some of the hardest words to say and one of the hardest things I have done. I know now, after several weeks off, work is not what I need at this time, and that doesn't make me a quitter. I need to be able to spend quality time with my husband, family, and friends. I need to take care of Loretta and her needs. And this I will do. Maybe this makes me a survivor. I know I will always have to struggle with cancer. It will always be a part of my life. But one day, God willing, there will be a cure for breast cancer and maybe in my lifetime. If not, I will still live my life, as we all should, with God's help, to the best of my ability one day at a time.

I asked a lady who was wheelchair bound because of Muscular Dystrophy, who had casts on both legs from breaking them at the knees, and who was taking chemo because her breast cancer had recurred after five years how she was able to handle things. She just smiled, such a beautiful smile, and said, "God just loves me a little more than some!" And I thought I had problems.

"God, I don't know why you want me to carry this load. I can see no good in it and it's awfully heavy. But, if you want me to carry it, I will."

Today, God smiled upon me.

Martha Falterman & Neppie Trahan & Loretta Schultz

About the Author

When Martha Falterman was diagnosed with cancer, her first thought was of her daughter, Toni. She was only sixteen years old and Martha wanted to see her grow up. She was the reason Martha fought this disease. In the last eight years, she has seen her daughter mature and grow up to be a fine young lady. "Thank you Lord."

Martha said, "Now I would have a second reason to battle this disease. My grandson, Logan, is the new 'love of my life.' When and if this cancer should return, I would fight it until my last breath. I want to see him grow up."

This is also dedicated to each of you that have been diagnosed with breast cancer and have the courage to fight. Each time I meet a new survivor and hear her story, I get new strength. To each of you, I say, "You are my heroes." Remember the greatest thing in the world is the ability to move in a positive direction.

Neppie Constantin Trahan lives in Lafayette, Louisiana with her husband, Freddy. They are both considered true Cajuns. Neppie loves good food, music, Cajun dancing, and visiting with family. The simple things are important to her and she considers every day a gift from God and what we do with it is our gift to Him.

Neppie said that when she was diagnosed with cancer, she needed hope. The books she found were all medical and she wanted to know how her life would change not just her health. She asked why didn't anyone write a book about emotions, family, and hope? Now finally, with Martha and Loretta, she did. According to Neppie, a second chance at life is our gift from God. This book is our gift to all of you who are going through cancer.

"Thank you to my daughters Shawn, Shannon, and Shelly and my grandchildren Hailey, Braden, and Garret for giving me the courage to live. I want to celebrate life. I feel my story is one of true love, from learning to love myself to sharing love with my husband, my best friend, while dealing with cancer."

Diagnosed with breast cancer five years ago, Loretta Schultz says that her love of life, family, and friends is what enables her to endure the things she must in order to fight the cancer inside of her.

Loretta has retired and is now limited to what activities she can do. Cancer and all the cancer treatments over the years have taken a toll on her body. But she still enjoys camping, fishing, photography, and the company of her family and friends.

According to Loretta, "This is a war. Too many soldiers have lost their battle. I vow to keep up the fight until there is a cure for breast cancer or I too lose the battle, which ever comes first."